DETOX YOUR BODY

A Holistic Approach to Health with the Wisdom of
Traditional Chinese Medicine

Foods, Massage & More

By Zhao Yingpan

SCPG

Text by Zhao Yingpan
Translation by Shelly Bryant
Design by Wang Wei

Editor: Cao Yue

ISBN: 978-1-93836-896-7

Address any comments about *Detox Your Body* to:

SCPG
401 Broadway, Ste.1000
New York, NY 10013
USA

or

Shanghai Press and Publishing Development Co., Ltd.
Floor 5, 390 Fuzhou Road, Shanghai, China (200001)
Email: sppdbook@sppdbook.com

Printed in China by Shanghai Donnelley Printing Co., Ltd.

1   3   5   7   9   10   8   6   4   2

CFP provides the image on page 148.

Contents

Preface

According to traditional Chinese medicine, the human body contains many toxins. A toxin is any substance that cannot be discharged quickly and has adverse effects on bodily systems, such as blood[1] stasis, phlegm-dampness[2], cold, indigestion, qi[3]

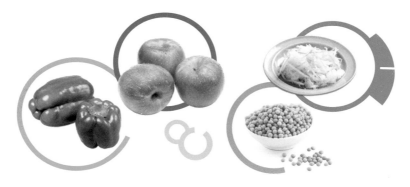

---

[1] The substance that is controlled by the pulse and circulates throughout the body. It is a red liquid with nutritional and moisturizing effects. Blood belongs to *yin*, so is also called *yin* blood.

[2] The name of an ailment, referring to a symptom of the bodily constitution, which is often caused by improper diet or disease. Phlegm here also refers to abnormal accumulation of bodily fluids, which is a pathological product. Dampness is either internal or external. External dampness refers to humidity in the air and living environment. It will invade the body and cause disease. Internal dampness refers to dysfunction of the digestive system, an uncontrollable flow of water in the body that leads to the accumulation of bodily fluids, or the accumulation of bodily fluids due to excessive dietary water, alcohol, cheese, and cold drinks.

[3] In TCM, qi is the subtle, fundamental substance that constitutes the body and maintains life activities. This term also includes physiological functions. In TCM terms, qi has different meanings when combined with other words.

stagnation (obstruction of the circulation of vital energy) and internal fire[4]. When they accumulate in the five *zang* organs (the heart, lungs, liver, spleen, and kidneys) these toxins accelerate the aging process of these organs, causing the skin, muscles, bones, and nerves they nourish to age at the same rate. Although they are hidden deep inside the body, toxins leave indications of their whereabouts on the surface in various forms such as hyperplasia and acne. It is important to identify where the toxins are hidden, and expel them from the body as quickly as possible.

Effective detoxification methods involve maintaining a regular diet and healthy living habits, as well as massage, diet therapy, and tea therapy recommended by TCM experts. If you make adjustments to your diet and follow the methods recommended in this book for a period of time, you will find that although you're not dieting, your body feels lighter. Although you're not having beauty treatments, your complexion is rosy, and although you're not taking supplements, your vitality is restored.

---

[4] A TCM term, meaning that the *yin* and *yang* of the body have lost balance and the endogenous fire is vigorous. "Fire" describes some hot symptoms in the body. Getting internal fire is also an internal heat syndrome that occurs with an imbalance of *yin* and *yang* in the body. Specific symptoms include red and swollen eyes, sores at the corners of the mouth, yellow urine, toothache, and sore throat. It is either "excessive fire" or "deficient fire." Excessive fire refers to the syndrome of excess heat due to hyperactive *yang* heat, which is mostly caused by the internal invasion of pathogenic fire-heat or the result of spicy food. Excessive mental stimulation and dysfunction of the visceral functions can be another cause. Deficient fire is mostly caused by internal injury and strain, such as long-term illness, depletion of vital energy, and excessive strain that leads to visceral imbalance and weakness, resulting in internal heat, which then turns into deficient fire.

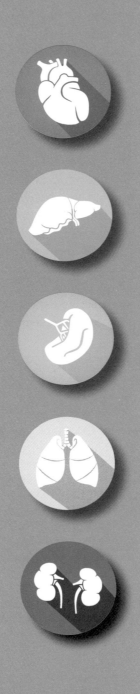

Chapter One
Knowing about the Toxins in Your Body

TCM and Western medicine have their own definition of "poison" or toxins. Although there are differences, there are also similarities. In TCM theory, "poison" includes an imbalance of *yin* and *yang* caused by the five endogenous evils, the six exogenous evils, internal injury caused by the seven emotions, as well as inappropriate diet, overwork, and lack of physical activity. The five endogenous evils refer to internal wind, cold, dampness, dryness, and heat caused by an imbalance of *yin* and *yang* and the *qi* and blood in the *zang-fu* organs; the six exogenous evils are the six external factors of wind, cold, summer heat, humidity, dryness, and fire that invade the body; internal injury refers to the seven emotional changes: joy, anger, anxiety, overthinking, grief, fear, and fright.

1. What Are Toxins?

TCM regards all ills as "poisons" or toxins. They can be divided into the following categories:

Heat toxins: When one's *yang qi*[1] is hyperactive, the body will produce heat toxins. Dry mouth, a bitter taste in the mouth, halitosis, swollen and bleeding gums, nose bleeds, dry and

---

[1] Anything, including movements, that are outward, possess the ability to rise upward, are hyperactive, light, or have functionality, and have *yang* attributes, which are opposite to *yin qi*.

hard stools, oily face, acne, and sweating hands and feet are the manifestations of this toxin.

Cold toxins: Opposite in nature from heat toxins, cold toxins can be divided into external and internal cold. While common colds and joint pains are a result of a cold wind invasion, which is an external factor, internal cold is caused by a deficiency of *yang* and a decline of viscera function, characterized by cold body and limbs, feeling cold in the lower back and abdomen, clear and colorless urination, and loose stools.

Fire toxins: When heat reaches its extreme, it becomes fire. In other words, when heat toxins reach a certain degree, they become fire toxins. Redness in the local area, swelling, heat, and pain are just mild symptoms of fire toxins. When it becomes severe, manifestations include fever, headache, irritability, scanty dark urine, constipation, red tongue with a yellow coating, as well as oral ulcers, and sores at the corners of the mouth.

Damp toxins: Damp is divided into external damp and internal damp. External damp is induced by a hot and humid environment, and manifests as rheumatic issues such as joint pain. Internal damp is caused by a weakness in the spleen and stomach, and poor transportation and transformation of foods and fluids[1] in the body. Malfunction of the spleen and stomach's transportation and transformation function can be caused by an inappropriate diet. When there is a deficiency in the spleen, vital qi[2] will be weakened, allowing the invasion of external damp, and hindering

---

[1] Fluid is the general name given to all normal bodily fluids. It includes the normal secretions of all viscera, gastric juice, intestinal juice, saliva, and joint fluid. It also includes urine, sweat, and tears in metabolites. Except for blood, all other normal fluids belong to the bodily fluid category.

[2] The general term for normal functional activities of the body and the various health maintenance abilities generated, including self-regulation, the ability to adapt to the environment, the ability to resist pathogens and diseases, and the ability to recover and heal.

the normal transportation and transformation function of the spleen and stomach. Manifestations of internal dampness are a loss of appetite, abdominal distension, diarrhea, loose stools, sallow complexion, edema, and a pale tongue with a moist coating.

Parasitic toxins: Parasitic toxins damage and erode local tissues, consuming nutrients and essence. Eating raw meat carries the risk of parasitic infection in the intestines and stomach. Symptoms of toxins from parasitic infection are abdominal pain, tooth grinding, sallow complexion, and poor digestive function. Skin symptoms such as scabies, ringworm, and ulcers can appear.

Toxins accumulated from food: The spleen and stomach are in charge of digestion, absorption, transformation, and transportation of food. If there is a dysfunction, food cannot be transformed and transported. This food will accumulate in the stomach. Over time it will turn into toxins, damaging the spleen and stomach, and causing symptoms such as loss of appetite, chest tightness, belching, acid regurgitation, poor stools, and acne.

Toxins from drugs: There is an old saying that there is a degree of poison in every drug. The symptoms of drug poisons are relatively complex, so the details will not be discussed in this book. However, they are all harmful to the liver. It is very important to have some knowledge of drugs and understand their toxicity and side effects.

Blood stasis toxins: Blood stasis toxins are the pathological product of abnormal blood function. If allowed to remain in the body, blood stasis will block meridians[3], preventing the body

---

[3] Meridians and collaterals are channels that transform and transport *qi* and blood, and connect the viscera with the body surface and all parts of the body. They are the regulatory system of the body's functions. The longitudinal trunk line contains the meridians, which are main channels for the movement of *qi* and blood around body. The branches that lead off from the meridians are called collaterals.

from being fully nourished by *qi* and blood. If this happens, various symptoms will appear, including stabbing pains throughout the body, pain at specific fixed locations, abnormal bleeding, and ecchymosis.

Toxins generated by emotions: Emotions generally refer to the seven kinds of emotional changes: joy, anger, anxiety, overthinking, grief, fear, and fright. These are the psychological reactions to external stimuli. In TCM, it is believed that emotions are generated by the gasification of the five *zang* organs. When a person's emotions are out of balance, harm can be done to their *zang-fu* and blood and *qi*, affecting their health. Too much joy can harm the heart; anger can harm the liver; overthinking can harm the spleen; grief can harm the lungs; and fear can harm the kidneys. Once emotions become excessive, they will harm the body.

The "poisons" or toxins in TCM are more abstract and broader than in Western medicine, where they are more specific and detailed. The following are some common toxins:

Biotoxins: Biotoxins, also known as natural toxins, are various substances produced by animals, plants, and microorganisms that are toxic to other organisms, such as the bite of a poisonous snake.

Toxicity and side effects of drugs: Most Western drugs are chemically synthesized, and have certain level of toxicity along with side effects. This is clearly indicated on the packaging. Because of their quick effect, Western medicines, especially antibiotics, tend to be abused. The over-use of antibiotics causes intestinal flora disorder, killing too many probiotics in the intestines. It also raises drug resistance in the body, preventing effective drug treatment in emergency cases.

Toxins caused by human factors: Human-inflicted toxins are wide ranging. Some examples are organophosphorus and organochlorine in pesticides, as well as carbon monoxide and ethanol. These toxins will cause a certain degree of damage once they enter the human body, and may even lead to death. One example is alcohol—a common toxin. Drunkenness is alcohol poisoning. Drinking a lot in one sitting will cause abnormalities to a person's physical functions, and can cause serious damage to the nervous system and liver. Within a few minutes of drinking, alcohol will reach the brain, reducing the function of brain cells and inhibiting the myocardium. The heart will have to accelerate its beats to adapt to this state. The first glass will make you feel relaxed. However, continued drinking will increase the alcohol concentration of the blood, affecting the brain's nerve center. Drinking can lead to extreme and violent behavior. Driving under the influence of alcohol often leads to car accidents because alcohol inhibits a person's ability to judge accurately and slows down their reaction time.

Toxins in food: This is the most common "poison" in daily life. Examples of such food are poisonous mushrooms, sprouting potatoes, and undercooked French beans. Although some foods contain toxins, not everyone will feel their effects. Firstly, the intake required to cause harm is different. Secondly, everyone's bodily constitution and response to toxins are different. Finally, some people are born more susceptible to allergic reactions. Even eating eggs and drinking milk may make them feel unwell. This group of people must be more cautious with their daily diet.

Toxins in the air: The main sources of PM 2.5 in haze are dust, coal combustion, biomass combustion, automobile exhaust, garbage incineration, industrial pollution, and secondary inorganic aerosols, all of which will undoubtedly cause harm to the body. Studies have shown that the harmful substances produced by house decoration are usually higher than harmful outdoor air pollutants. To reduce the concentration of harmful indoor substances, proper ventilation is needed over a prolonged period.

Toxins in drinking water: Water pollution is a result of domestic sewage and industrial wastewater. Drinking polluted water will cause symptoms such as nausea, diarrhea, vomiting, and headaches, and in serious cases may even cause cancer.

Toxins in daily items: Things that we use daily such as perfume, shaving cream, toothpaste, soap, shampoo, laundry detergent, nail polish, and cosmetics contain chemicals that can penetrate the body through the skin and produce toxins.

2. Are There Toxins in Your Body?

In addition to the external factors that people are aware of, the human body itself also produces toxins. The "waste" produced by the body's metabolic activities needs to be removed promptly, or it will have a great adverse impact on the body.

Accumulated fecal matter in the colon: Constipation is the result of trapped feces that have not been excreted from the body. Some people who suffer from this issue also experience insomnia, irritability, disturbed sleep, and depression. Diet therapy can alleviate these conditions. However, when symptoms such as bloody stool, anemia, emaciation, fever, black stool, and abdominal pain occur, you should go to a hospital for treatment.

Uric acid: Uric acid is the waste product of metabolism, and is excreted through urination. If the level of uric acid is too high, or there is a weak flow of urine, excess uric acid will be deposited in the body's soft tissues or joints, causing inflammation. To prevent this, drink more water, eat more vegetables such as eggplants, lettuce, and celery, and cut down on your consumption of red meat (that is, meat that is red before cooking, such as pork, beef, and mutton).

Free radicals: A small number of free radicals is good for the human body, as they can protect it from invasion by foreign substances such as chemicals. However, free radicals are the main factor in aging. Excessive free radicals increase oxidative stress leading to skin pigmentation, allergies, and cardiovascular issues. They also accelerate the aging process. The way to eliminate free radicals is to eat more fruit and vegetables that are rich in anti-oxidants, such as broccoli, carrots, corn, asparagus, cauliflower, and kiwi fruit.

Cholesterol: When cholesterol is mentioned, conditions such as hypertension, coronary heart disease, cardiovascular occlusion, and obesity come to mind. However, cholesterol is not always a toxin. As a structural component of the body, it is also the precursor for the biosynthesis of many important substances. However, if cholesterol deposits become excessive, then the consumption of red meat and eggs should be reduced. Instead, eat more corn, carrots, kelp, and apples.

Triglyceride: This name may sound unfamiliar, but when ailments like cerebral thrombosis, coronary heart disease, and kidney disease attributed to dyslipidemia are mentioned, many will nod their heads in recognition. As high triglycerides do not show specific symptoms, it is important that middle-aged and elderly people take regular physical health checks at a hospital. If the triglyceride level is high, it is advisable to cut down on the consumption of food containing a lot of starch and sugar. If the levels of both triglycerides and cholesterol are high, strict control must be exerted over your diet and weight.

Lactic acid: Pain, fatigue, and lethargy after physical activities and exercise are linked to a build-up of lactic acid or lactate in the body. When too much lactic acid has built up, the muscles will contract, squeezing the blood vessels, blocking blood flow, and inducing muscle pain, chills, headaches, and heaviness in the head. To alleviate this discomfort, make sure you get enough high-quality sleep, perform light stretching exercises, and eat more foods rich in B vitamins.

Edema: Edema is linked to viscera such as the lungs, spleen, and kidneys. In addition to the damp toxin mentioned in TCM, edema can also be attributed to an external invasion from wind pathogens[1] (see footnote on page 16), internal invasion of sore-toxins, inappropriate diet, long-term illness, and fatigue. The most common forms of edema are lower limb edema, menstrual edema, pregnancy edema, and kidney edema, with edema obesity as the most common disease, seen in people who get fat just by drinking water. According to TCM theory, edema is divided into *yang* edema and *yin* edema. *Yang* edema is characterized by the rapid spread of edema from the eyelids and head to the whole body. The swollen skin on the affected area becomes tight and shiny, and bounces back quickly when pressed. This condition is accompanied by symptoms such as frequent thirst, deep color and difficulty in urination, and constipation. To alleviate *yang* edema, it is necessary to disperse the inhibited lung *qi* to relieve superficies syndrome[2]. *Yin* edema is characterized by whole-body edema, loose stools, and non-deep color nor difficulty in urination. A good way to improve this condition is to warm and tonify the spleen and kidneys.

Mental toxins: Stress, depression, confusion, distress from prolonged periods of working overtime, and exam nerves are common mental states. These negative emotional conditions lead to tension and repression, causing symptoms such as decreased immunity, endocrine disorders, and metabolic disorders. Mental toxins can be eliminated by self-regulation, eating cereals and grains, consuming fruit and vegetables, eating less greasy and irritating food, and going out for a walk.

If there is a buildup of toxins in the body, changes will take place physically and emotionally. Let's do a self-check. Do you need to detoxify?

---

[1] A pathogenic factor caused by wind. Along with cold, summer heat, humidity, dryness, and fire, it is one of the six exogenous pathogens. It is a pathogen with the characteristics of positive movement—rising, upward, outward, prone to attacking the muscle surface and making the body leak gas and liquid. Its pathogenic characteristics come on rapidly and change frequently. The pain moves around the body, and is aggravated by the wind, mostly affecting the upper part of the body.

[2] Illness that has not attached the vital organs of the human body.

Check Yourself for Toxins

1. Irregular wake-up time, and weak limbs.

2. Heavy hair loss; hair is dry with split-ends.

3. Large, soft abdomen, like a swimming ring.

4. Weak lower back and knees, frequent urination, forgetfulness, and inability to stay focused.

5. Acne-prone skin, especially on the forehead.

6. Often out at social gatherings; an increasingly obvious "beer belly."

7. Losing temper easily over trivial matters.

8. Constipation; only defecating once every two or three days, sometimes accompanied with bleeding.

9. Insomnia or disturbed sleep.

10. Feeling tired and sleepy in the morning.

11. Bad breath that is not resolved by brushing teeth.

12. Poor digestion; food that you used to like does not appeal to you anymore.

13. Declining immunity; prone to flu.

14. Dull, rough, and often itchy complexion.

15. For women, less blood flow during periods; short or irregular menstrual cycle, dark in color.

Result:

1–3 items: In good shape. Just make slight adjustments to your work-rest schedule.

4–6 items: Slightly poor physical condition. Be more aware, and carry out simple detoxification.

More than 6 items: Your body is overwhelmed. Strictly modify your lifestyle and habits, and engage in comprehensive detoxification.

You can also find out whether you have toxins in your body, and their location, by observing your face.

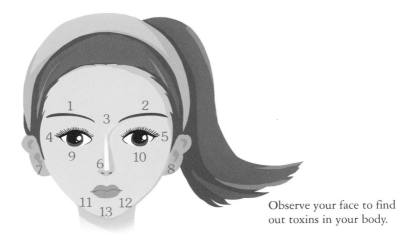

Observe your face to find out toxins in your body.

Zones 1 and 2: Take note when acne or red swelling begins to appear on your forehead. It is time to adjust your mood, because it may be an indication of a heart problem. Reduce your consumption of junk food and fatty meat, and eat more healthy food to alleviate your acne.

Zone 3: Acne and itching in the middle of the forehead often indicate heart and liver problems. Drinking, staying up late, and stress can aggravate symptoms; instead, eat less greasy food and have enough rest.

Zones 4 and 5: Darkened facial complexion, eye bags, edema under the eyes, and a deepening of crow's feet signify that the kidneys are overloaded. Eat a plainer diet, nourish your liver, and consume more black sesame, beans, and bean products.

Zone 6: When pimples appear on the tip and wings of the nose, it signifies excessive hyperactive heart heat. If your nose bleeds and the blood is bright red, it may be an indication of lung heat. Consuming food with heat eliminating properties will improve your condition.

Zones 7 and 8: The ear is a representation of the health condition of the kidneys. If the auricle turns red or purple, it indicates poor renal blood circulation. When this happens, drinking should be reduced. Eat more grains and take more exercise to encourage blood circulation.

Zones 9 and 10: Itchy, swollen cheeks can be induced by problems in the respiratory system. Fresh air and food that soothes the throat, moistens the lungs, and generates bodily fluids can help improve this condition.

Zones 11 and 12: Acne breakouts and oily skin are indications of abnormal hormone levels in the body. Make sure you get enough sleep, drink more water, and eat more vegetables. Women should keep warm during menstruation, drink warm water, and nourish and restore the health of their liver, stomach, and spleen.

Zone 13: Acne and itching on the chin signifies that there is a problem in the digestive system. Consume more food that nourishes the stomach, such as millet, pumpkin, and yam.

3. How to Get Rid of Toxins?

The following questions carry important information that will help you understand more about detoxification so that you can carry it out more effectively.

Can drinking water help to remove toxins? The answer is "yes." Drinking water can stimulate gastrointestinal peristalsis and help you defecate. It can also regulate water in your body and accelerate sweating, achieving detoxification. However, when using this method to detoxify, there are important points to consider. First, it is advisable to drink warm water, as cold water can cause gastrointestinal discomfort. Second, avoid drinking too much water. If too much water is taken in, the body must discharge the excess, diluting the salt in the blood. This will reduce the body's absorption ability, allowing some water to be absorbed into the cells, causing tissue edema. In serious cases, it may also cause water poisoning, dizziness, thirst, and fainting.

Is menstruation a form of detoxification? Every month following the first menarche, women will go through the physiological process of menstruation to stimulate the body's hematopoietic function, self-regulation, and self-improvement. Menstruation is a means of detoxification in which the necrotic and exfoliated endometrium is discharged with menstrual blood, readying the uterus for the next cycle. Like sweating and defecation, menstruation encourages metabolism, "cleaning up" the uterus every month.

Can eating vegetables help to detoxify? While the nutrients in vegetables have no detoxification effect, they have other functions such as anti-aging and promoting digestion. In TCM, vegetables can be used to detoxify, and the effects are positive. For example, spinach can nourish the *yin* and subdue the *yang* of the liver; bitter gourd can eliminate heat and fire; cucumber can improve detumescence and diuresis, and winter melon can invigorate the spleen and remove dampness.

Is a vegetarian diet the only way to detoxify? Although there are many benefits of a vegetarian diet, such as weight control, disease prevention, beauty and skin care, it is not an absolute. Nutritional imbalances such as iron deficiency and lack of animal protein can occur from eating only vegetables. A healthy detoxification plan requires a balanced diet, with both meat and vegetables. A proper diet together with a healthy lifestyle can achieve better results.

Which type of food has the greatest detoxifying effect? It is not realistic to assume that eating one kind of food can remove all the toxins in the body. Cereals, fruits, and vegetables are good ingredients for detoxification and health.

For which groups of people is detoxification not suitable? People with weak constitutions are advised not to undergo detoxification. They will need to consult a doctor or another medical professional to restore their health. Another group of people who are not suitable for detoxification are the elderly who are in a poor physical condition, as it may affect their normal rest and recuperation. The next group are people suffering from severe gastroenteritis and hemorrhoids. They will need to seek a doctor's advice and treatment. Pregnant women belong to a special group, as whatever they do is related to the health and safety of their babies. If issues such as constipation, edema, spots, and stretch marks occur during pregnancy, diet therapy can help alleviate them. Cold and stimulating food should be avoided. After they have given birth, women should not be in a hurry to recover their figure through detoxification, but should be recuperate under the guidance of doctors.

TCM diet therapy detoxification. TCM perceives the human body as a "small universe" in which the organs are interrelated, forming a unified whole. The five *zang* organs (the heart, liver, spleen, lungs, and kidneys) have the following corresponding relationships with the five elements: metal, wood, water, fire, and earth.

The kidneys belong to the water element. They govern the bones and filter the blood.

The liver belongs to the wood element, and is in charge of immunity and detoxifying.

The heart belongs to the fire element, and is the power pump that transports the blood around the body.

The spleen belongs to the earth element; while the stomach holds the water, the spleen absorbs the water and provides it to the whole body.

The lungs belong to the metal element, and are responsible for breathing, inhaling oxygen and exhaling carbon dioxide.

The properties of metal, wood, water, fire, and earth correspond to the colors and flavors of food. By understanding the properties of the corresponding elements of the five *zang* organs, it is possible to identify which foods are beneficial to these organs.

The flavor associated with the water element is salty, and the

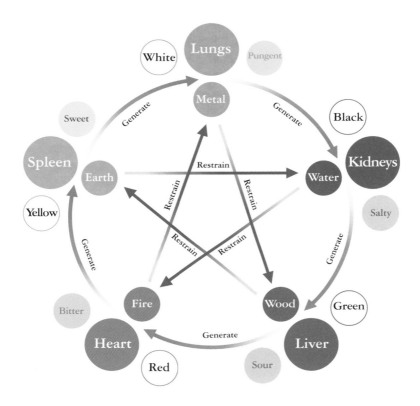

The relatiouships among the five *zang* organs, the five elements, and the food flavor and color.

food color is black. Subsequently, black food corresponds to the kidneys and bones. Eating such foods more frequently can help the metabolism related to the kidneys, bladder, and bones to work normally, preventing the accumulation of excess water that causes edema. It also strengthens the bones.

The flavor associated with the wood element is sour, and the food color is green. Green food enters the liver; when added to the daily diet, it can nourish and protect the liver. Spinach, broccoli, asparagus, and chrysanthemum coronarium are examples of common green foods.

The flavor associated with the fire element is bitter, and the food color is red. To nourish the heart, eat some red food. Red gives a feeling of warmth and heat. It corresponds to the color of the blood and the heart, which is responsible for blood circulation. People with pale complexions and cold limbs should eat more red food.

The flavor associated with the earth element is sweet, and the food color is yellow. The spleen and stomach are nutrient providers in the body. Only when these two organs are nourished and well can *qi* and blood be strong. Common yellow foods rich in carotene and vitamin C can strengthen the spleen and stomach, such as bananas, millet, and pumpkin.

The flavor associated with the metal element is pungent, and the food color is white. Food corresponding to the lungs is mostly white, with a cool, calm temperament. It can clear and strengthen the lungs, encourage gastrointestinal peristalsis, enhance metabolism, and make the skin more elastic and lustrous.

The above information is just the tip of the iceberg in TCM healthcare. In the subsequent chapters, we will explain the use of TCM diet therapy and tea therapy, supplemented by massage and daily habits to detoxify the five *zang* organs and restore the health and lightness of the body.

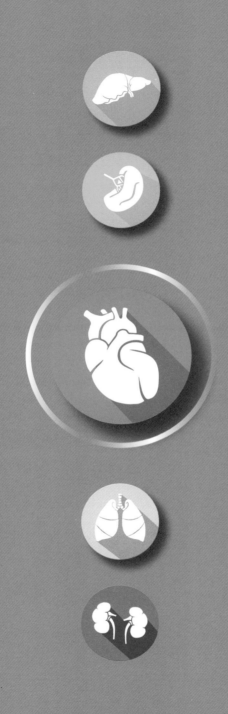

Chapter Two
Detoxifying the Heart

Among the five *zang* organs, the heart belongs to the fire element. It relies on the rise of the *yang* to nourish and vitalize all parts of the body. If a person lives to be 100 years old, they would have experienced around four billion heartbeats in their life. Therefore, if you want to live longer, you will need a strong heart.

In TCM theory, the heart governs the blood and vessels[1]. It is both the start and end point of blood circulation. It is the driving force and center of the circulatory system, as it beats day and night, sending blood to the blood vessels, circulating, and supplying oxygen and nutrients to the body. The function of the heart governing the blood and vessels relies on the heart *qi* to push, as well as the sufficiency of the blood and the smoothness of the blood vessels. Only when the heart *qi* is strong and abundant can the blood operate and circulate normally in the blood vessels. To sum up, the three prerequisites for maintaining the function of the heart governing blood and vessels are abundant *qi*, enough blood, and smooth blood vessels.

A TCM practitioner makes a diagnosis through the sensory perceptions of "observing, listening, asking, and feeling." "Feeling" constitutes taking the pulse, and is also known as pulse diagnosis. When the heart governing blood and vessels is functioning normally, the pulse is gentle and powerful, beating

---

[1] The heart *qi* drives the blood to move with the pulse, flowing around the body, circulating endlessly, and providing nutrients and moisture.

in a uniform rhythm at a moderate rate that is neither fast nor slow. However, if the heart governing blood and vessels is functioning abnormally, pulse diagnosis will often detect diseases related to a slow heart rate or fast heart rate. The heart governs mental activities[1], referring to the emotional center of the body. The heart's functions of governing blood and vessels and governing mental activities are interrelated, and affect each other. The heart governing the blood and vessels is controlled by the heart *shen* (state of mind). The heart rate, the speed of blood flow, and the contraction and relaxation of blood vessels are often affected by factors such as emotions. Meanwhile, due to the fact that the mind and spirit rely on nourishment from the heart blood, insufficient blood supply and low spirits will cause symptoms such as becoming dazed, forgetfulness, insomnia, and excessive dreaming.

Modern life is full of pressures. Setbacks, blows, and emergency situations affect a person's emotional state, making them depressed, and leading to issues with sleeping and eating. Some people bounce back quickly, regaining confidence and hope. Some recover slowly, and take longer to emerge from dejection. When one is free from anxiety and burdens, and is always cheerful, living a long life is a definite possibility. This is because mental activities are controlled by the heart.

In general, only when the heart is well can one have enough blood and *qi*, energy, and good spirits. It is the "elixir" for a long life.

---

[1] High-level central nervous activities such as spirit, consciousness, and thinking, which are presided over by the heart. The heart governs mental activities: This is one of the most important functions of the heart. If the function of the mind dominating mental activities is normal, then the spirit is vigorous and clear. However, if there is a dysfunction, it can lead to mental disorders, such as palpitations, forgetfulness, insomnia, and mania, and can also cause functional disorders of other viscera.

1. Are There Toxins in Your Heart?

The importance of the heart is common knowledge. Before any obvious cardiac abnormality manifests itself, check for the following symptoms to see if your heart is "poisoned."

Tongue ulcers: Tongue ulcers of all sizes are very common. Some have a burning sensation while others are itchy, and they often recur. TCM practitioners believe that the tongue and the heart are the most closely related organs, so when an ulcer appears on the tongue, it usually indicates that there is "fire" or "fire poison" in the heart. It should be noted that there are two common diseases that are similar to the symptoms of "heart fire." The presence of small blisters around the mouth is known as herpetic stomatitis, while dry cracks in the corners of the mouth are a symptom of canker sores.

Changes to the tongue coating: The coating on the surface of the tongue is a thin, evenly-spread white layer, slightly thicker in the middle and at the root of the tongue. When the body is experiencing health problems, the thickness of the tongue coating will change. If the tongue is red and the coating is not obvious, it indicates deficient heart fire. If the tongue coating is thick and yellow, it indicates there is excessive heart fire, and this is often accompanied by yellow urine and dry stools.

Forehead acne: The forehead is managed by the heart. When excessive heart heat becomes toxic, there will be a breakout of acne on the forehead. For example, during exam season, staying up late can lead to excessive anxiety, which in turn results in breakouts of acne on the forehead. People who work under high pressure and often do overtime also experience breakouts of forehead acne. However, not all cases indicate heart problems. People who are bad tempered, angry, fussy, and competitive are prone to this as well. Acne symptoms are more obvious in summer. People with heart heat and acne must make an effort to regulate the inside and outside of their body. They should avoid irritant foods such as spicy and greasy dishes, and say no to stimulating beverages like strong tea and coffee. They should eat more fruit and vegetables, maintain good living habits, avoid staying up late, and make sure they get enough rest and sleep. Daily exercise can accelerate blood circulation and metabolism to help dispel toxins from the body.

Insomnia and palpitations: The causes of insomnia are many, including drinking coffee in the day and being unable to sleep at night, and an irregular work and rest schedule. Some people who face great psychological and emotional pressure tend to lie awake at night, unable to switch off. A heartbeat that is too fast, too slow, or irregular can cause palpitations. Insomnia and excessive dreaming are related to insufficient blood and the absence of emotional support, which are manifested as a weak physique, pale complexion, palpitations, and forgetfulness. Insomnia is due to excessive heart fire leading to dry mouth syndrome, which is usually caused by excessive internal heat or liver *qi* stagnation[1] that has turned into heat. In addition, a shock or surprise can cause harm to the heart, leading to restlessness and then palpitations, insomnia, irritability, a dazed state, and even mental disorders with symptoms such as crying and laughing without apparent reason, talking incessantly, mania, and madness.

Chest tightness and stabbing pains: Feeling out of breath, short of breath, unable to exhale, or feeling pressure on the chest are all manifestations of chest tightness. More serious is a stabbing pain. These symptoms are usually brought about by negative emotions such as depression and unhappiness. People who are more sensitive tend to harbor negative emotions when

---

[1] Stagnation of liver *qi* is mostly caused by emotional depression and obstruction to *qi* movement. The liver has the function of relieving *qi*, and likes to rise and release. If the liver is injured due to emotional discomfort or anger affecting the rise and release of *qi*, it will cause liver stagnation.

they encounter unpleasant situations, resulting in chest tightness and stabbing pain.

2. Habits That Harm the Heart

The heart is the most important of the five *zang* organs. It is the master of life, yet is very fragile and easily harmed. The following are some common forms of negligence that cause damage to the heart.

Overwork: There are two aspects that lead to overwork. The first aspect is physical exhaustion. This could be due to the huge physical strain when the workload is too heavy, or if the duration of work is too long. Another example is going beyond the limit of one's physical strength when exercising. The body is not able to get enough rest to recover, and will eventually break down from accumulated fatigue. The second aspect is over-straining the body when it is weak or has not recovered after an illness. This will also suffer the same consequence as the former—a physical breakdown that will lead to illness. Similar to the healthcare of the five *zang* organs, the heart *shen* should be allowed to rest and recuperate, and the liver *qi* needs to be unobstructed. In daily life, release and relieve emotional stress to avoid causing over exhaustion to the heart *shen*. The consequence of overworking the body consumes the *qi* of the body. Mental fatigue is often caused by excessive loss of heart *qi* and heart blood. Commonly seen symptoms such as restlessness, fatigue, dry mouth, dry throat, ulcers on the mouth and tongue, palpitations, and chest tightness are the manifestation of deficiency fire[2], which is the consequence of mental fatigue.

Excessive cold: The heart is a *yang* viscera, belonging to the

---

[2] Compared with "excessive fire," it is characterized by deficiency hyperactivity due to physical weakness, kidney *yin* deficiency, or kidney *yang* failure.

element of fire, and governs blood. The flow and circulation of blood depend on the warmth generated by the heart *yang*[1] and the driving force of the heart *qi*. Consequently, in TCM, it is believed that among the six external factors which cause diseases, the greatest threat to the heart is *yin* cold. Any cold stimulation will make the blood vessels contract and spasm to varying degrees, causing insufficient blood and oxygen in the tissues, and greatly increasing the secretion of catecholamines in the body, resulting in increased blood viscosity, platelet aggregation, and thrombosis. When the body encounters cold air, reflexive coronary artery contraction will occur, resulting in myocardial ischemia and angina (chest pain). If this continues for a long time, it will lead to acute myocardial infarction (heart attack).

Excessive mental stimulation: The human spirit is the most closely related to the heart among the five *zang* organs. Unrestrained joy and anger can stimulate symptoms such as an accelerated heart rate, elevated blood pressure, shortness of breath, sweat secretion, or even shock or fainting, as well as other abnormal conditions in severe cases. To avoid over-stimulation of the spirit, be adept at regulating your emotions, as our mental and emotional states can be managed. In TCM theory, the heart governs happiness, the lungs govern sorrow, the spleen governs thinking, the liver governs anger, and the kidneys govern fear. Subsequently, our emotions are closely related to the health of the five *zang* organs. Too much joy affects the heart. The heartbeat becomes irregular, and the mind is unable to stay focused, even to the extent of losing sanity.

Frequent excessive sweating: Relying on air conditioning over long periods is not good for the health. However, excessive sweating will also damage your heart, leading to deficiency in the body. Moderate sweating, that is, sweating without dripping,

---

[1] The *yang qi* of the heart, in contrast to the heart *yin*, is the excitable driving force and warm side of the heart.

is the healthier form of perspiration. However, if the amount of sweating exceeds the physiological compensation limit of bodily fluids and blood, it will deplete them. The body's *yang qi* is the driving force for the operation and management of sweat secretion. Excessive sweating will drain *qi,* injuring both the *qi* and blood, and leading to the loss of nourishment from the heart and causing distress to mental activities. This results in dizziness, palpitations, shortness of breath, mental fatigue, insomnia, and oliguria (low urine output). Profuse sweating injures bodily fluids and blood, and drains *yang qi*. Summer is regarded as the best season to conserve *yang*. However, with excessive sweating, the body's *yang* will be over-exploited.

3. Massage Therapy to Detoxify the Heart

There are twelve meridians distributed symmetrically in the body. They are the Taiyin Lung Meridian of Hand (LU), Jueyin Pericardium Meridian of Hand (PC), Shaoyin Heart Meridian of Hand (HT), Yangming Large Intestine Meridian of Hand (LI), Shaoyang Sanjiao Meridian of Hand (TE), Taiyang Small Intestine Meridian of Hand (SI), Yangming Stomach Meridian

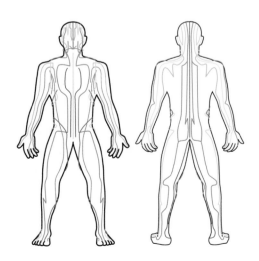

Main meridians on the body. Front (left) and back (right).

of Foot (ST), Shaoyang Gallbladder Meridian of Foot (GB), Taiyang Bladder Meridian of Foot (BL), Taiyin Spleen Meridian of Foot (SP), Jueyin Liver Meridian of Foot (LR), and Shaoyin Kidney Meridian of Foot (KI). Among them, Shaoyin Heart Meridian of Hand is closely related to the heart. Therefore, any abnormality occurring in the viscera (heart and small intestine) connected with the meridian or the part it runs through is seen as an ailment of the heart meridian. A few minutes of massage on the Shaoyin Heart Meridian of Hand every day can solve heart problems.

Press the Xinshu Acupoint[1]

On the posterior torso lies the Taiyang Bladder Meridian of Foot (BL). There is a group of very special points called *shu xue* (acupoints) on it. It is the part where the *qi* of the Du Meridian (governor vessel) passes through the Taiyang Bladder Meridian of Foot and infuses into the internal organs, and also where the *qi* of each internal organ reaches the surface of the body. Those infused into the heart are called Xinshu acupoints.

In the meridians, the acupoints have two main roles. First, they can be used as the basis for diagnosis, as diseases can be detected by pressing on these points. Second, the corresponding visceral diseases distributed in the chest area can be treated by stimulating the acupoints located on the back.

In TCM, mental and emotional abnormalities such

---

[1] The surface of the body is closely connected with deep tissues and organs, and communicates with them. There are acupoints dotted all over it. Rather than isolated points, they are places where nerve endings are dense, or points that thicker nerve fibers pass through. According to TCM, they reflect the infusion of *qi* and blood into and out of the viscera, meridians, and collaterals. They can be regarded as the reaction points of disease, the stimulation points of treatment, and the sensitive points for beauty. Therefore, they form the basis of acupuncture and massage.

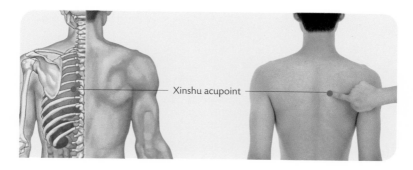

Xinshu acupoint

as insomnia, forgetfulness, irritability, speech difficulties, cardiovascular disorders like chest tightness, palpitations, arrhythmia, and angina pectoris, plus problems such as hyperhidrosis, spontaneous sweating, night sweating, pale complexion, and dull skin, are related to the heart. Treatment can be performed at the Xinshu acupoints. Gently massage them for several minutes with the pulp of your thumb or index finger. Deep pressure and strong stimulation are not recommended.

Acupoint location: On both sides of the back. Under the spinous process of the fifth thoracic vertebra on the posterior torso, 1.5 cun from the posterior median line.

Massage method: Press the Xinshu acupoints with the pulp of the index finger. The manipulation should be gentle. Massage for two minutes each time.

Press the Shaohai Acupoint

The Shaohai acupoint belongs to water in the five elements, and the heart belongs to fire. According to the principle of mutual nourishment and mutual restraint among the five elements, fire is restrained by water, so by stimulating the Shaohai acupoint to remove heart fire and nourish kidney water, heart heat can be alleviated and treated.

In addition, the causes of modern diseases are changing from a single natural factor to a combination of social and psychological factors. New personality deviations, behavioral abnormalities, mental disorders, and physical and mental

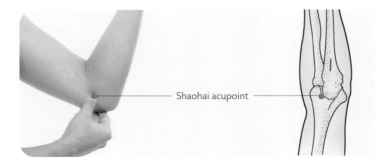

Shaohai acupoint

illnesses are constantly emerging. TCM perceives many of these to be related to excessive heart fire. To encourage mental health, massage the Shaohai acupoint to dispel heat and eliminate desire.

Acupoint location: On both arms. In the anterior part of the elbow, on the horizontal line, at the anterior edge of the medial epicondyle of the humerus.

Massage method: Press the Shaohai acupoints with your thumb in the morning and evening, for 1 to 3 minutes each time.

Knead-Press the Laogong Acupoint

The pericardium is the protective tissue that shields the heart from direct invasion of external pathogens. At the same time, the pericardium is the outward transportation channel of the heart *qi* and blood, so the relationship between the two is very close, and their functions overlap.

Perform this action frequently: Cross your hands and rub your palms repeatedly. This is where the very important heart-protecting Laogong acupoint is located. Issues that can be cured include bad breath, a bitter taste in the mouth, a dry mouth caused by too much heart fire, mental and emotional abnormalities caused by anxiety, palpitations, chest tightness, and pain caused by a blockage in the heart vessels.

Acupoint location: On both hands. In the palmar region, at the horizontal proximal end of the third metacarpophalangeal joint, close to the third metacarpal bone between the second and third metacarpal bones.

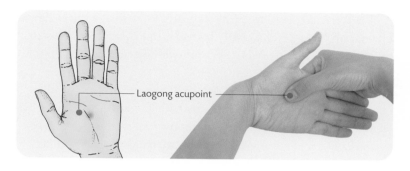

Laogong acupoint

Massage method: Knead-press the Laogong acupoints for 1 to 3 minutes each time.

4. Diet Therapy to Detoxify the Heart

To eliminate heart toxins and dispel heart fire, you must first distinguish whether there is a deficiency or excess, and then identify its root cause. High fever, headache, red eyes, a thirst for cold drinks, irritability, constipation, yellow urine, a red tongue with yellow coating, and nose bleeds indicate excessive fire[1]. Eat more bitter food to dispel heart heat. If your throat is dry and painful, your cheekbones are red, your mind is irritable, and your sleep is affected, this indicates deficiency fire. When clearing the heart of toxins, nourish the kidneys, reduce unnecessary sweating, and protect bodily fluids, so as to moisten the heart *yin* and blood.

Bitter Food

Excess heart fire not only causes irritability and insomnia, but also leads to other ailments. The first thing to do is to clear heart fire. The safest way to do this is through diet therapy instead of medication. This is beneficial to health, and can also prevent diseases.

---

[1] Excess syndrome caused by the hyperactive fire pathogen.

"Bitter-cold" food in TCM is mostly food with a bitter flavor, but not all bitter food actually tastes bitter. Bitter food consists mainly of household vegetables and wild vegetables, such as celery, luffa, bitter gourd, and celtuce.

Celery: This vegetable is rich in dietary fiber, and it can encourage peristalsis in the intestines. Celery also contains chemicals that encourage fat decomposition, which can reduce the absorption of fat and cholesterol, with a detoxifying effect.

Luffa: Luffa has the functions of detoxification and dispelling heat. It contains a chemical known as saponin, which has a strong cardiac strengthening effect and can enhance the function of the myocardium.

Bitter gourd: This vegetable is effective at detoxification and beautifying the skin, and can remove pathogenic heat, relieve fatigue, cleanse the heart, and clear the eyes.

Celtuce: This vegetable has a fresh and slightly bitter taste. It can stimulate the secretion of digestive enzymes, and is effective at detoxification and dispelling internal heat.

Consuming more bitter food can help patients with excessive heat dispel this toxin. However, consuming too much can damage the stomach *qi* and reduce bodily fluids, especially for patients who have deficiency fire. According to the TCM principle of nourishing *yang* in spring and summer, food that induces warmth is better for your summer diet. If it induces too much cold, it will encourage dampness and produce phlegm, trap the spleen, and damage the *yang*. Therefore, when purging heart fire, we must keep the balance of *yin* and *yang*, according to the environmental climate and our physical conditions.

Red Food

TCM holds that red is fire and *yang*, which is connected to the heart, so red food can enter the heart and blood when consumed. For people with insufficient heart *qi* and weak heart *yang*, red food will be very beneficial. Many red foods have strong antioxidant properties and anti-aging effects, and at the same time provide protein, minerals, and vitamins to enhance the function of the heart and *qi* and blood.

However, the consumption of red food in animals should be reduced, because red meat such as beef, mutton, and pork is rich in fat and high in calories. Prolonged period of overeating such foods is likely to lead to a hardening of blood vessels, an increase in blood pressure, and abnormal blood lipids and blood viscosity, ultimately endangering the health of the heart. If you wish to eat meat and also want to nourish your heart, you should eat less meat and more vegetables. Balanced nutrition is the cornerstone to health. Common red foods such as red beans, longans, and red dates can be added to stews and porridge for extra nourishment.

Red beans: These are very effective at dispelling internal dampness by clearing the small intestines. They facilitate urination and detumescence, and remove stagnant water in the body, thereby detoxifying and reducing swelling.

Longans: Longans are sweet, and are good for the heart and spleen, replenishing *qi* and blood. Regular consumption has a tonic effect on the body.

Red dates: These are also a good health tonic. Eating more of them can improve vitality.

Red drinks consist of black tea and red wine. After black tea has been fully fermented, dried, and processed, the polyphenol content is greatly reduced, but the theaflavin content increases. Theaflavin regulates blood lipids and prevents cardiovascular disease. Red wine contains the antioxidant resveratrol, which can reduce cholesterol. Drinking a small glass of red wine every day is good for the heart. That is the reason why the rate of cardiovascular disease in France is much lower than that of other countries.

Delicious Healthy Recipes
Bitter Gourd Omelet
Ingredients: 150 g bitter gourd, two eggs, coriander, garlic, and salt to taste

Method: ❶ Mince the garlic. Wash the bitter gourd, and slice thinly. Blanch the bitter gourd slices with salt water, then drain them. ❷ Add salt to the eggs and beat. Add bitter gourd slices, and mix well. ❸ Heat a little oil in a pan. Pour in the bitter gourd and egg mixture. Fry over a low heat until both sides are golden. ❹ Turn off the heat, cut the omelet into small pieces, and garnish with coriander and minced garlic.

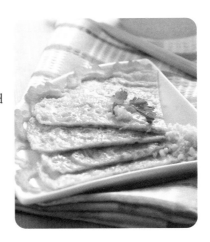

Effects: TCM holds that bitter gourd omelet can relieve summer heat. It has a good therapeutic effect on common symptoms such as acne, blistering in the mouth, and mouth ulcers, and is able to help the body detoxify.

Celtuce Rice Porridge

Ingredients: 30 g celtuce, 50 g round grain rice, salt to taste

Method: ❶ Peel, wash, and cut the celtuce into small pieces. Wash the rice. ❷ Put the celtuce pieces and rice into a pot. Add an appropriate amount of water to boil. ❸ Cook until the rice is soft and the juice is starchy. Add salt and cook for a while.

Effects: People suffering from palpitations and insomnia should eat more celtuce because it is rich in potassium. Eating it frequently can reduce atrial pressure, eliminate tension,

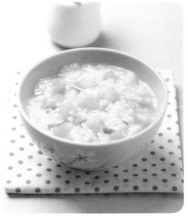

and improve sleep. People who prefer a lighter taste can stir fry the vegetable. However, it is not advisable to make it into a cold dish, as the cold nature of the celtuce may hurt the stomach.

White Fungus and Pea Sprouts

Ingredients: 50 g white fungus, 100 g pea sprouts, cooking wine, starch, and salt to taste

    Method: ❶ Soak the white fungus in warm water, wash it, then blanch it in boiling water. Remove. Wash the pea sprouts, blanch them in boiling water, and then remove. ❷ Add water to the pot. Add cooking wine, salt, and white fungus, and cook for three minutes. ❸ Thicken with starch, stir fry, and dish up. Garnish with pea sprouts.

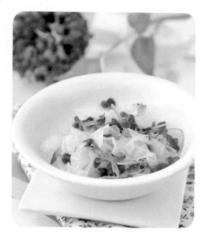

    Effects: Eating peas frequently can reduce the triglycerides in the body and lower the incidence of heart disease. Pea sprouts taste good and have high nutritional value, and are particularly suitable for women and children.

Winter Melon, Kelp, and Barley Soup

Ingredients: 200 g winter melon, 50 g kelp, 30 g barley, salt

    Method: ❶ Wash and shred the kelp. Wash the barley. ❷ Wash and skin the winter melon, and cut it into thin slices. ❸ Put the barley, kelp, and winter melon into the

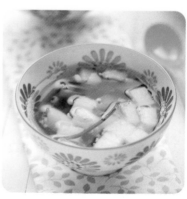

pot together, and add an appropriate amount of water to boil.
❹ Simmer over a low heat for about half an hour, and season
with salt.

Effects: Winter melon can relieve swelling and heat.
This soup can strengthen the spleen, and has a diuretic effect,
reducing water retention; it can also support weight loss and
beautification.

Almond Soy Milk

Ingredients: 50 g soy beans,
10 g almonds, 5 g pine nuts,
rock sugar

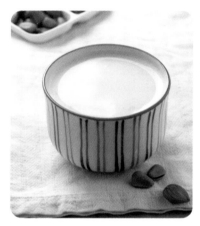

Method: ❶ Soak the soy
beans for ten hours. Remove
and wash. ❷ Put the soy beans,
almonds, and pine nuts into a
soy milk machine. Add water
and press the start button.
(If the soybean machine does
not have a cooking function,
steam the soy beans, almonds,
and pine nuts beforehand.) ❸ After it is done, filter it. Add an
appropriate amount of rock sugar; mix, and stir.

Effects: The amygdalin in almonds can prevent heart attacks
and help maintain normal blood pressure. In addition, the rich
vitamin E in almonds can purify the blood and delay the aging
process. They are very good for maintaining women's health.

Lily Bulb Congee

Ingredients: 30 g fresh lily bulbs, 50 g round grain rice, rock
sugar

Method: ❶ Separate the sections of the fresh lily bulbs and
wash them. Wash the rice. ❷ Put the rice in the pot with an
appropriate amount of water, and boil it at a high heat. ❸ Lower
the heat and continue to cook. When it is almost cooked, add

the fresh lily bulbs and rock sugar, and cook until it is starchy.

Effects: High levels of stress, insomnia, and palpitations are all manifestations of heart toxins. Eating lily bulbs can alleviate internal heat and dryness, uplift the spirits, and keep negative emotions and anxiety at bay.

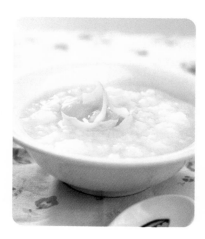

Fried Beef with Sweet Pepper

Ingredients: 200 g sweet pepper, 100 g beef tenderloin, egg, cooking wine, starch, ginger, soy sauce, broth, sweet sauce, salt

Method: ❶ Crack the egg and separate the egg white. Wash the beef tenderloin and cut it into shreds. Add salt, egg white, cooking wine, and starch, and mix well. **❷** Wash

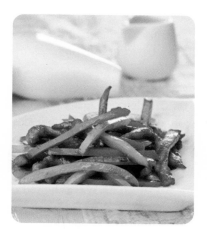

and shred sweet pepper and ginger, and set aside. To make the sauce, add soy sauce and starch to broth, and set aside. **❸** Stir fry the shredded sweet pepper until it is 80% cooked, then set aside. Stir fry the beef, then add sweet sauce, sweet pepper, and ginger. Stir fry until fragrant. Thicken with the sauce that was just made, and stir fry evenly.

Effects: Beef nourishes the *qi* and blood, strengthening the spleen and stomach. It is suitable for people with anemia, blood deficiency, and weak physique.

Wolfberry Rice Paste

Ingredients: 60 g round grain rice, red dates, wolfberries, ginger

Method: ❶ Wash the rice and soak it in water for two hours. ❷ Wash the wolfberries and soak them in warm water. ❸ Wash the red dates and remove the pits. Cut the ginger into pieces. ❹ Put all the ingredients into the soy milk machine, and add water. Start

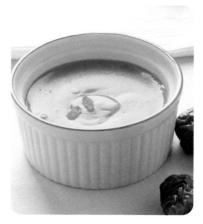

the machine to make rice paste. Dish out when it is done, and garnish with a few wolfberries. (If the soybean machine does not have a cooking function, steam the rice beforehand.)

Effects: Wolfberries can calm the nerves and replenish deficiencies. It is a high-quality food for menopausal women, as it can detoxify heart poison and replenish *qi* and blood. For stomach cold[1], more ginger can be added to warm it.

Ginger Jujube (Red Date) Tea

Ingredients: 10 g ginger, 10 g red dates, 20 g brown sugar

Method: ❶ Wash the red dates and remove the pits. Shred the ginger. ❷ Put the red dates, shredded ginger, and brown sugar into the pot, and add water to boil. ❸ Decoct the soup, and drink it twice a day.

Effects: This diet therapy recipe invigorates the spleen-stomach and replenishes *qi*[2]. It can also prevent colds, resist

---

[1] When the stomach is attacked by cold pathogens, or when cold or raw food is eaten, this can lead to pathological changes such as a deficiency of *yang qi* and an excess of *yin* cold in the stomach.

[2] The treatment of *qi* deficiency in the spleen and stomach using medicines that invigorate *qi*, strengthen the spleen, and balance the stomach.

influenza viruses, improve women's symptoms such as cold abdominal pain, and strengthen weak *qi* and blood. People with chapped lips, dry mouths, and dysphoria with a feverish sensation in the chest, palms, and soles[3] have fire hyperactivity due to *yin* deficiency[4], and should not use this recipe.

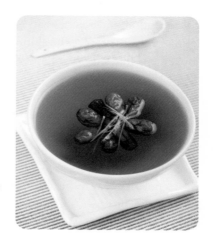

Steamed Egg with Tomato

Ingredients: one tomato, one egg, salt

Method: ❶ Wash, peel, and dice the tomatoes. Fry them in a pan over a high heat for a while. ❷ Add salt to the egg, and beat it. Add an appropriate amount of water to the egg mixture, and steam it over a low heat. ❸ When the eggs are about 70% cooked, add the diced tomatoes and continue steaming.

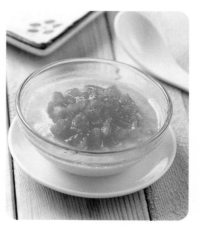

Effects: The vitamin C and vitamin P in tomatoes have an anti-aging effect, and protect the blood vessels. Regular

---

[3] Self-awareness of the manifestations of fever in the palms of both hands and feet and chest, which can be accompanied by restlessness and rising temperature.

[4] Pathological change of hyperactive deficiency fire when there is a *yin* deficiency, and *yin* cannot control *yang*, leading to excessive *yang*.

consumption of tomatoes can remove freckles, delay the aging process, protect the skin, help digestion, improve bowel movement for defecation, and dispel toxins.

Longan and Lotus Seed Porridge

Ingredients: 80 g round grain rice, 10 g longans (without pits), ten lotus seeds, rock sugar

    Method: ❶ Wash the lotus seeds and soak for two hours. Soak the longans in warm water for five minutes, and pour away the impurities. Wash the rice.

❷ Pour the lotus seeds, longans, and rice into the pot. Add an appropriate amount of water, bring to the boil, and add rock sugar. Turn to a medium or low heat and continue to stew for 90 minutes.

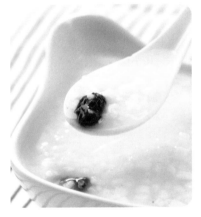

    Effects: Longans are good for the heart and spleen, replenishing *qi* and blood, and calming the mind. In addition, they also have a therapeutic effect on palpitations and neurasthenia.

Red Date Porridge

Ingredients: 30 g round grain rice, six red dates

    Method: ❶ Wash the rice and red dates. ❷ Put the rice and red dates into the pot. Add an appropriate amount of water. ❸ Bring to boil over a high heat. Turn down the heat and boil until it becomes

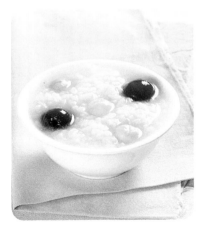

porridge.

Effects: Red dates are good for nourishing the body, *qi*, and blood. Eat them to enhance vitality, resist the invasion of toxins such as exogenous pathogens, and enhance the body's immunity. Women with anemia can add two or three red dates to rice, soup, or porridge every day to improve their condition.

Peanut Sweet Potato Soup

Ingredients: one sweet potato, one cup of fresh milk, peanuts and red dates

Method: ❶ Wash the peanuts and red dates and soak them for 30 minutes. Wash, peel, and cut the sweet potatoes. **❷** Put the peanuts, sweet potato, and red dates into the pot, and add an appropriate amount of water. **❸** Boil over a low heat until the sweet potato softens. Turn off the heat. **❹** Dish up the soup and add fresh milk.

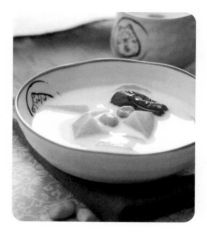

Effects: When eaten often, sweet potato can help reduce cholesterol, prevent toxin deposits in the body, and prevent atherosclerosis. It reduces the incidence of cardiovascular and cerebrovascular diseases.

Celery and Pineapple Juice

Ingredients: ½ stalk celery, ¼ pineapple, salt

Method: ❶ Wash and cut

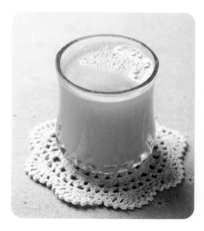

the celery into small pieces. ❷ Remove the pineapple skin, cut the fruit into small pieces, and soak it in salt water. ❸ Put the celery and pineapple into the juicer. Add an appropriate amount of water and start the juicer.

Effects: Celery tastes sweet and pungent. It has a calming effect, and can clear heat, detoxify, and reduce blood pressure. For people with insomnia, celery is a sleep enhancing food. Using this vegetable in salads or a quick stir fry will reduce the loss of nutrients.

White Radish and Lotus Root Juice

Ingredients: 100 g lotus root, 100 g white radish, honey

Method: ❶ Wash the white radish and lotus root, cut, and put in the juicer separately. ❷ Mix the two juices together, add honey, and mix well.

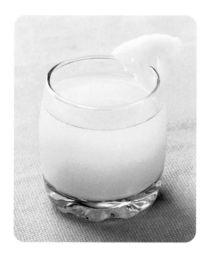

Effects: Lotus root dispels heat to eliminate emotional frustrations, cool the blood, stop bleeding, and disperse blood and stasis. People with epistaxis, blood stasis, hematemesis, and bloody stool will benefit from eating it.

5. Tea Therapy to Detoxify the Heart

Tea is very good for a variety of health conditions. Whether green or black, it is the preferred beverage for detoxification. In recent years, herbal flower tea has become very popular among young women. It can improve the appearance and uplift the mood. Take good care of the heart, the skin will have a rosy glow, adding charm to your appearance.

Rose Tea

Ingredients: rose, rock sugar

Method: ❶ Put the rose buds and rock sugar in a teapot together. Pour in hot water at about 80℃ (leave water that is boiled at 100℃ to stand for a few minutes). ❷ Cover it, let it sit for five minutes. Drink.

Effects: Drinking rose tea often can encourage blood circulation in the body, help the body dispel blood stasis and toxins, and alleviate the symptoms of feeling depressed and abdominal pain during menstruation.

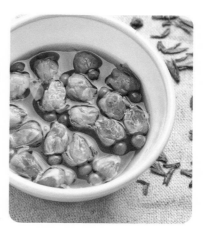

Rose Ginseng Tea

Ingredients: eight rose buds, five slices American ginseng, three red dates

Method: ❶ Wash the dates. ❷ Put the dates, rose buds, and American ginseng into a teapot. Pour in hot water at about 80℃. ❸ Cover the teapot. Leave it to sit for five minutes before drinking.

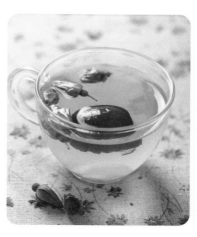

Effects: Drinking rose tea with some American ginseng encourages blood circulation; it can replenish *qi* and nourish *yin*, expelling heat and generating bodily fluids.

Rose Milk Tea

Ingredients: six rose buds, one cup milk, raisins, wolfberries

Method: ❶ Put the rose buds, raisins, and wolfberries into

a teapot. Pour in hot water.
❷ Add milk after five minutes.
Mix evenly and serve.

Effects: Rose milk tea is
the top choice for beauty and
keeping the skin moist. It can
be drunk at any time, especially
two hours before going to bed,
as it can help sleep.

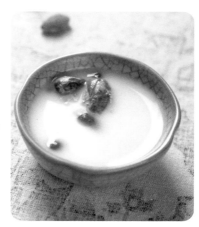

Roselle Tea

Ingredients: five roselle
blossoms, honey

Method: ❶ Put roselle
blossoms into the pot. Add an
appropriate amount of water.
Bring to boil. ❷ Turn off the
heat after three minutes. Leave
it soaking in the pot for about
five minutes. ❸ Strain and
pour tea into a cup. Add honey
to taste.

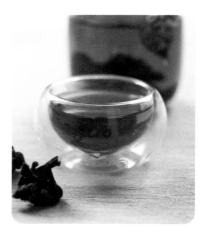

Effects: The roselle flower
is a good antioxidant food as it
contains a lot of anthocyanins,
which can effectively eliminate
free radicals in the body. It is good for detoxifying and
beautifying, and very good for delaying the aging process.

Roselle Chrysanthemum Tea

Ingredients: eight roselle blossoms, ten chrysanthemum
blossoms, rock sugar

Method: ❶ Put roselle, chrysanthemum and rock sugar
into a teapot together. Pour in hot water. ❷ Keep it covered for
about ten minutes. Stir evenly. Serve.

Effects: Modern research has found that roselle can reduce cholesterol and triglyceride in the body, and can prevent and treat cardiovascular diseases. This tea is also suitable for people who are suffering from anxiety, insomnia, and disturbed sleep.

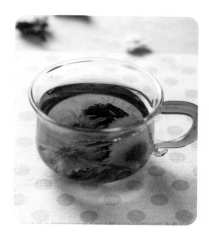

Wolfberry Longan Tea

Ingredients: two rose buds, four longans, wolfberries

Method: ❶ Remove the outer shells of the longan. Add this to a cup with the wolfberries. Pour in hot water. ❷ Add rose buds after ten minutes and let it stand for a little while. Consume when it is ready.

Effects: A lot of people make a habit of staying up late. As time goes on, their skin will become dull, and dark circles will begin to appear under

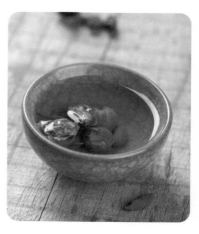

their eyes. When this happens, it is time to detoxify the heart and liver, to restore blood circulation to normal. Drinking this tea regularly can nourish *yin* and enhance beauty. It can improve various symptoms caused by staying up late, and can restore the skin.

Wolfberry Red Date Tea

Ingredients: five red dates, ten wolfberries, rock sugar

Method: ❶ Remove the pits of the red dates. Put the red

dates into a pot with the wolfberries. Add water and bring to the boil. ❷ Add rock sugar after five minutes. It is ready when the rock sugar has fully dissolved.

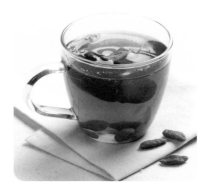

Effects: When there is insufficient heart blood, symptoms like becoming dazed, forgetfulness, insomnia, and disturbed sleep will begin to manifest. Only when the blood is replenished can the spirit be refreshed. Regular consumption of wolfberries, red dates, and red beans can nourish the blood, and the spirit will naturally be lifted.

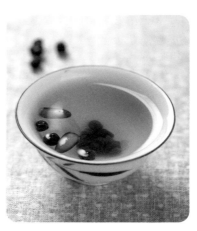

Schisandra Chinensis (Five-Flavor Fruit) and Pine Nuts Tea

Ingredients: Schisandra chinensis, pine nuts, honey

Method: ❶ Put the schisandra chinensis in a cup, pour in boiling water. ❷ Keep it covered for five minutes. Add the pine nuts and honey. Stir well.

Effects: Schisandra chinensis can nourish the five *zang* organs and calm the heart *shen*. It is good for the elderly and patients with heart disease.

Red Date Beauty Tea

Ingredients: ten red dates, appropriate amount of black tea leaves and sugar

Method: ❶ Remove the
pits of the dates. Put them in
the pot with the sugar. Add
water and bring to the boil.
❷ Pour hot water onto the tea
leaves, and keep it covered for
five minutes. ❸ Mix the tea
and red dates soup, stir evenly.

Effects: Red dates are
one of the best foods for
detoxification and anti-aging,
and can prolong life. They also
tonify deficiency in *qi*, nourish
the blood, and calm the nerves,
and can relieve symptoms such
as insufficient *qi* and blood,
fatigue, and weakness.

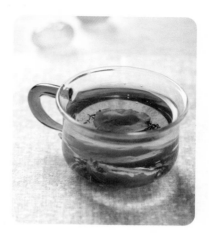

Red Date and Raisin Tea
Ingredients: five red dates,
15 raisins, black tea

Method: ❶ Remove the
pits of the dates. Put them
into a pot with the raisins. Add
water and bring to the boil.
❷ Put in the black tea and
brew for another three minutes.

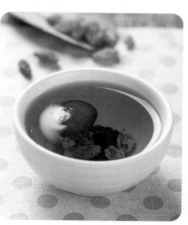

Effects: Women with irregular periods are prone to mild
anemia, with symptoms such as facial pallor, listlessness, and
cold hands and feet. A handful of raisins a day can be eaten as
a snack as well as diet therapy. In addition to supplementing
blood, raisins help to improve problems such as a dark yellow
complexion caused by insufficient *qi* and blood.

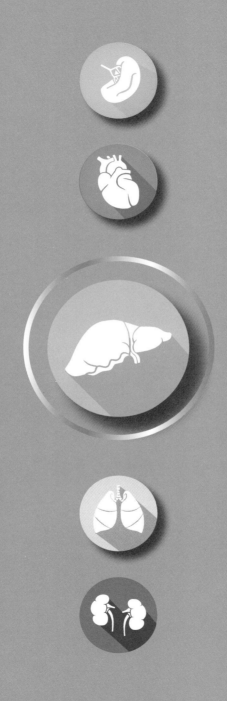

Chapter Three
Detoxifying the Liver

Among the five *zang* organs, the liver corresponds to the wood element. Wood is associated with plants in nature, growing freely without any restrictions. To nourish the liver, we should maintain a calm and happy mood and retain the organ's normal purification function. People nowadays find it difficult to do so, because there are a lot of pressures in daily life, as well as socializing. Drinking too much, staying up late, and over-indulgence in food can burden the liver to its limit. People become irritable. Whether they lose their temper or bottle up their emotions, over time, many health issues will arise, such as menstrual disorders, dizziness, and feeling thirsty but having no desire to drink water.

One of the most important functions of the liver is to release stagnated energy and clear blockages to ensure smooth flow. Many women are susceptible to mood swings, as well as being irritable and tiring easily, especially before and after menstruation. This is because women are blood-governed and liver-based. During pre-menstrual and menstrual periods, the liver's *yin* blood mostly concentrates in the uterus. As *yin* blood discharges, *yang qi* rises, causing transverse dysfunction of liver *qi*[1], resulting in the woman getting angry and losing her temper. This brings up the major function of the liver, which is to store blood. If the blood storage function of the liver is damaged, the body will tire easily, as blood supports the viscera, meridians, and limbs. Insufficient

---

[1] The pathological changes of liver failure, *qi* stagnation, and liver *qi* distortion invading the spleen and stomach.

liver blood will significantly reduce the blood flow to the whole body, thus affecting the delivery of oxygen and nutrients, and resulting in fatigue due to hypoxia and malnutrition.

"Anger" is not a morbidity, but is the manifestation of the nature of the liver. If the liver *qi* does not ascend and descend when it is supposed to, it can only indicate that the liver's purification function is abnormal. If you always suppress your emotions and often feel depressed and unhappy, there is a high likelihood that you will develop stagnation of liver *qi* that can cause obstruction to its normal function. So if you are unhappy, try to release your anger appropriately. On the other hand, if you are often angry, your liver *qi* will rise too much, and this will lead to dangerous symptoms such as hematemesis, fainting, and cerebrovascular hemorrhage. Meanwhile it is very important to remain calm, placid, and serene for the health of your liver *qi*.

1. Are There Toxins in Your Liver?

The liver is the most important detoxification organ in the human body. Liver cells contain abundant enzymes. Any drugs, hormones, or toxins produced by microorganisms, or endogenous or exogenous toxic substances rely on the liver to break them down so as to reduce the accumulation of toxins in the body. If the toxin cannot be discharged smoothly from the liver, the body will respond in many ways as a prompt.

Hyperplasia of the mammary glands: Even when people eat grains and cereals, they can also be affected by foreign invaders, such as drugs. Over time, toxins will accumulate in the body. The liver is the detoxifying organ responsible for cleaning up and expelling toxins and ensuring the health of the body. When the toxin level is too high and the liver is overburdened, some of these toxins will remain in the liver and become hepatotoxins, causing major damage to the body. In women, this will produce breast hyperplasia and destroy breast cells. Therefore, TCM treatment of breast hyperplasia focuses on clearing blockages in the liver and nourishing it. In TCM, it is believed that women are blood-governed and liver-based, as liver stores blood and is responsible for releasing stagnated energy. Therefore, when women get angry, there will be stagnation of the liver *qi*, leading to blood stasis; the liver meridian passes through the breast, so the breast is prone to swelling, pain, and hardened lumps.

Eye discomfort: In TCM theory, the liver opens at the eyes[1]. When there are problems with the eyes, patients will experience symptoms such as dry eyes, pain, or sensitivity to wind, all related to the liver. Dry eye syndrome is caused by insufficient liver blood and *yin* deficiency of the liver and kidneys[2]. Thus, we should nourish the liver and the kidneys. Red veins in the eyes may be caused by insufficient sleep or internal heat. Pain and swelling of the eyes accompanied by dizziness and headache may be caused by liver fire and internal heat.

Prone to depression and irritability: The liver is the organ responsible for regulating emotions. For this reason, when the liver has problems and toxins accumulate, an obstruction will arise to the transformation and transportation of *qi*, subjecting the patient to depression, feeling downcast, being short-tempered, and experiencing a range of negative emotions. When people feel depressed, they will be in an unhappy mood, which can cause a stagnation of *qi*. Therefore, the areas where nutrition remains in the body are the locations of the various *qi* stagnations, indicated by swelling and pain. To nourish your liver, first regulate your emotions. Include more oats, milk,

---

[1] The meridians of the liver are connected to the eye system, and the objective visual function depends on the release of liver *qi* and the nutrition of liver blood. The physiological and pathological conditions of the liver can be reflected in the eyes.

[2] A pathological change caused by deficient fire disturbed internally as *yin* is not able to control *yang*, and deficient *yin* fluid in the liver and kidneys leading to a lack of nurturing of the physique, internal organs, and the seven apertures in the human head.

bananas, fish, to your diet, as they can help improve your mood.

Vertical ridges on the nails: When your nail surface is not smooth and vertical lines begin to show, this may indicate that you are not getting enough rest. These vertical ridges will become more obvious when you physically overwork yourself, overuse your brain, or have insufficient sleep. If these ridges persist, it can be a sign of a lack of vitamin A in your body. Meanwhile, it is necessary to make adjustments to your regular schedule and go to bed earlier. Eat some foods that are good for the liver, such as pig liver, chicken liver, cauliflower, and carrots. Ridges on the nails are an indication of liver *qi* stagnation. People who are emotionally sensitive and fragile in spirit can develop liver *qi* stagnation more easily. To prevent this, keep warm, be happy, and get enough rest.

Palmar erythema (reddening of the palms): In patients suffering from chronic hepatitis, especially when liver cirrhosis has occurred, the skin shows patchy congestion at the thenar of the thumb and little finger, or red spots and rashes that turn pale when pressed. This is called hepatic palm or liver palm. To determine whether this indicates a problem with the liver, the patient's drinking and metabolic history will need to be reviewed, followed by a physical examination, liver function examination, ultrasound, and CT scan of the liver. What is the cause of liver palm? The body produces estrogen, which travels through the whole system in the blood. After performing its duty, it enters the liver to complete its decomposition and deactivation. If the liver function is abnormal, a large amount of estrogen will accumulate in the body, stimulating capillary congestion and expansion, and leading to palmar erythema.

2. Habits That Harm the Liver

Modern people live a fast-paced life. Their eating habits are affected, and irregular and unbalanced meals plus overeating can weaken the spleen and stomach and jeopardize the transformation and transportation function of these organs. In addition, factors such as mental tension, mood fluctuation, insomnia, and staying up late contribute to liver *qi* stagnation, transforming into fire and causing the transverse dysfunction of liver *qi*.

Overuse of the eyes: Mobile phones, computers, and televisions have become an increasingly inseparable part of life, work, entertainment, and leisure. Staring at a screen for a long time may hurt the eyes, but in actual fact, it is the liver that is ultimately harmed. Over-tiring the eyes will deplete a lot of liver blood. TCM states that to protect or nourish the eyes, the first thing is to replenish and nourish the liver and blood. If there is insufficient liver blood, or a deficiency of bodily fluids, or weak liver *qi*, the *yin* blood will not be able to reach the head, meaning that the eyes cannot get nourishment and moisture. When this happens, dizziness, dryness, and blurred vision will occur. People who use their eyes a lot need to protect their liver and nourish their blood. Include animal livers such as pig liver and chicken liver, into your diet, and supplement foods rich in vitamins such as beef, crucian carp, spinach, and shepherd's purse. In traditional Chinese medicine, Angelica sinensis and white peony can replenish blood, while chrysanthemum and wolfberry can brighten the eyes.

Excessive drinking: People tend to think that drinking is fine as long as they avoid getting drunk, not realizing that harm has already been done to their liver. It is true that the liver can detoxify, but this is not its only function. Its other jobs include promoting the transportation and transformation of the spleen and stomach, and ensuring the secretion of bile and excretion of metabolites. When wine enters the body, the alcohol in the wine will cause severe damage to the liver cells. It will disrupt the normal metabolism of the liver, and can cause alcoholic hepatitis and cirrhosis. Furthermore, according to TCM, because the liver meridian passes through the genitalia, drinking a large amount of alcohol will also affect sexual and reproductive functions.

Therefore, for the sake of one's own health and that of future generations, it is better to drink less. If you have to drink, it is advisable to stay on the safe baseline for healthy drinking, which is less than 40 g (alcohol) per day for men. The safe amount of alcohol consumption established medically is determined according to the body's metabolic capacity for alcohol. The maximum amount of alcohol that a normal adult body can break down each day is not more than 150 g.

Often staying up late: TCM views sleep as a very important way for the body to restore the balance of *yin* and *yang*. It is life's best energy saving method in its metabolic activities. In nature, *yin* dominates quietness and in turn, quietness generates *yin*, and abundant *yin qi*[1] encourages sleep. *Yang* dominates active energy and in turn, active energy generates *yang*, and abundant *yang qi* encourages wakefulness. Therefore, during rest and sleep, *yin* blood will return to the liver, and by laying still, the liver *qi* can be moistened. As a result, *yin* and *yang* will be in equilibrium, and the patient will feel calm and serene. However, if you often stay up late and don't get enough sleep, the blood *yin* will be channeled outward to the other parts of the body, and the liver will be unable to store blood. As a result, *yang qi* in the liver will be restless, leading to a variety of health issues such as flaring up of liver fire[2] and ascending hyperactivity of liver *yang*[3]. From 1:00

---

[1] The opposite of *yang qi*. *Yin qi* refers to the internal, downward, suppressed, weakened, and heavily turbid *qi*.

[2] Blazing liver fire ascends through the meridians and attacks the top of the head; it is the pathogenic change that occurs when there is a surge of *qi* and blood in the meridians.

[3] *Yang qi* of the liver. It dominates the ascent and release, in contrast with liver *yin*. Ascending hyperactivity of liver *yang*: A series of symptoms caused by the weakened astringent function of insufficient liver *yin*, allowing the liver *yang* to disturb the top of the head and eyes. The main symptoms are swelling and pain on the head, irritability, and weakness of the lower back and knees.

a.m. to 3:00 a.m., the *qi* and blood in the liver and gallbladder meridians are the most abundant, making this the best time to nourish the liver blood. It is also the time when the liver begins its detoxification. However, for liver detoxification to be carried out, you will have to be in a deep sleep. Some studies have shown that blood flow to the liver decreases by 40% when the body is in an upright position, 80%–85% while exercising, and ample in a supine position.

Over-medication: It is a well-known fact that the liver has a powerful detoxification function, and its metabolic activity is the most vigorous in the body. This is because the liver is able to break down, reduce, and diminish harmful substances that go into the body such as food additives, alcohol, medicines, smoke, and dust, to prevent them from causing damage. However, if you always over-medicate, you will eventually work the liver beyond its limit. Medication includes medicines that prevent illnesses, as well as supplements and tonics to encourage wellness, enhance beauty, and lose weight. However, all drugs have toxicity to some degree. Even prescribed drugs need to be metabolized and detoxified through the liver first. When too much medicine is taken, the liver gets very tired, leading to a decline in function. When two or more drugs act at the same time, the "double blow" may be hard for the liver to withstand. The damage of many drugs to the liver is not obvious when used individually. However, if they are used with other drugs, the impact on the liver may become greater, increasing the probability of damage. Therefore, do not take medicine unless you are sick.

3. Massage Therapy to Detoxify the Liver

Massage therapy can be used according to your individual condition, whether it is liver *qi* stagnation, hyperactive liver heat, rising liver *yang* of excess syndrome[1] (see footnote on page 60) or a deficiency of liver blood, or a deficiency of the liver-*yin* and kidney-*yin* of deficiency syndrome[2] (see footnote on page 60).

Press-Knead the Ququan Acupoint

When the body experiences symptoms of insufficient liver blood such as dizzy spells, blurred vision, palpitations and tinnitus, insomnia and disturbed sleep, weak lower back and knees, numbness of fingers, low menstrual volume, and flaccidity of the lower limbs, or if you often stay up late for a period of time, use your eyes too much, causing damage to your liver blood, you can apply the press-knead manipulation gently on the Ququan acupoint with your fingers. Massaging the Ququan acupoints of both legs often can clear blockage and stasis in the liver, and can effectively prevent and treat breast hyperplasia.

Acupoint location: On both legs. In the knee, the medial end of the popliteal stria, at the depression of the inner edge of the semitendinosus tendon.

Massage method: When applying the press-knead manipulation, you can use your fingers on the inner side of the knee, press-knead both the left and right acupoints in an upward direction for several minutes.

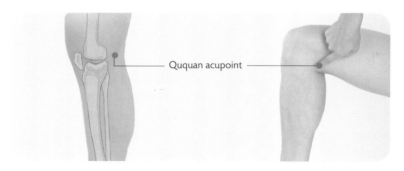

Ququan acupoint

---

[1] A syndrome represented by excessive pathogenic *qi*. It is caused by the stagnation of phlegm, water dampness, blood stasis, and food accumulation in the body due to the feeling of external pathogens or the dysfunction of internal organs. It is the opposite of deficiency syndrome.

[2] Weak syndrome caused by deficiency of vital *qi* and decline of visceral function.

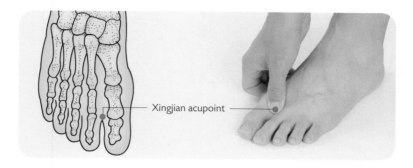

Xingjian acupoint

Massage Xingjian Acupoint

According to TCM, the liver meridian is distributed in both ribs, and the nipple belongs to the liver. Women are more emotional. They are prone to emotional fluctuations and anger, that can easily lead to liver *qi* stagnation, poor blood flow, chest tightness, breast pain, irregular menstruation and other discomforts of the body. These symptoms are especially more apparent before menstruation. During this time, the liver *qi* loses its moisture and goes up to the breast. The symptoms of breast pain become more obvious. When the above symptoms appear, massage the Xingjian acupoints. This is good for clearing blockage and stasis, cleanse liver and purge heat. Women can massage this point often to regulate *qi* and blood, dredge meridians and collaterals, relieve pain, as well as alleviate headache, tinnitus, deafness and insomnia.

Acupoint location: On the dorsum of both feet, between the first and second toes, at the junction of the red and white skin.

Massage method: Press the Xingjian acupoints with the pulp of your thumb, exhale, you will feel a slight pain. Repeat this action for three minutes.

Press-Knead the Taichong Acupoint

Getting angry and feeling dissatisfied is something everybody experiences. The right way to do when this happens is to make sure your anger has a way to be let off and dispelled. From TCM study of the meridians, you will be pleasantly surprised at

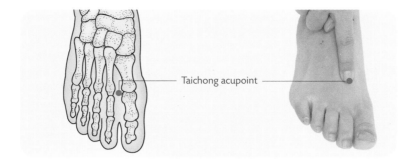

Taichong acupoint

the unexpected effects if you can press your Taichong acupoint at this time. Any disease of the liver meridian, whether it is liver heat, liver *yang*, liver *qi* or liver wind, it can be treated by purging, smoothening and eliminating. In TCM, it is believed that the reason why people are irritable and experience emotional disorder is because the flow of liver *qi* is obstructed. Massaging this point by pressing can help release stagnated energy, eliminate anger and regulate emotions.

Acupoint location: In the dorsum of both feet, between the first and second metatarsal bones, in the front depression of the metatarsal base junction.

Massage method: Press-knead the Taichong acupoints with the pulp of your index finger for three minutes every day. This method is very effective at eliminating anxiety.

4. Diet Therapy to Detoxify the Liver

Needless to say, the most important thing to do for nourishing the liver is to regulate the emotions. In terms of diet according to TCM, you can eat some food that cleanses and replenishes the liver, so as to reduce its burden appropriately.

Cold Nature Food and Sour-Sweet Food

The most commonly used food in diet for purging liver fire is mainly foods with cold properties, which can also clear away the heart fire. The common symptoms of headaches, a bitter taste in the mouth, increased eye discharge, irritability, and impulsivity are mostly caused by the flaring up of liver fire, brought about by excessive fire. This should be treated with purgative methods. However, dizziness, hot flushes and night sweats, weakness and tenderness in the lower back and knees, insomnia, and disturbed sleep are mostly caused by *yin* deficiency of the liver and kidney, brought about by deficiency fire. This should be treated with tonifying methods.

TCM theory states that to clear and purge excessive fire in the liver, whether it is medicinal treatment or diet therapy, products should be mainly of a bitter-cold properties or sweet-cold properties, such as chrysanthemum indicum, bitter gourd, and mung beans. To nourish the kidney water and liver blood, use products that are mainly salty-cold, sweet-cold, and sour-sweet in properties, such as watermelon.

According to TCM, sour flavor enters the liver, and has the functions of restraining, arresting discharge, and stopping perspiration and diarrhea. Modern clinical studies have found that sour food can enhance digestive function, protect the liver, lower the blood pressure, and soften the blood vessels. Pomegranate, hawthorn, and orange are examples of sour foods. Because spicy and sweet flavors can stimulate *yang* to create heat, patients with hyperactive liver fire should try to avoid eating spicy, fried, fatty, rich, warm and heat-inducing, greasy, and damp foods. Sweet-sour foods can transform *yin* and generate bodily fluids, so eating more sour and slightly sweet tasting foods, such as strawberries, tomatoes, and black plums, will be beneficial as they will help transform bodily fluids, replenish *yin* and blood, and reduce deficiency fire.

Green Food

The liver governs green foods, and sour flavors tonify the liver. Therefore, green foods are more nourishing to the liver. They contain a large amount of dietary fiber, which can encourage peristalsis in the stomach and intestines, and help the excretion of metabolites in the body, thus reducing the burden of the liver. In this way, it indirectly plays a role in protecting the liver.

Green food enters the liver meridian, and often plays the role of the body's scavenger and guardian, clearing heat and detoxing, removing obstructions in the liver and strengthening it. Moreover, it can reduce and eliminate the damage caused by various toxins, while enhancing immunity and alleviating fatigue. Examples of green foods are broccoli, chrysanthemum coronarium, mung beans, spinach, and green pepper.

Broccoli: Rich in vitamins, carotene, and minerals. Its ascorbic acid can enhance the detoxification function of the liver.

Chrysanthemum coronarium: This vegetable is often eaten in spring. It has high nutritional value, and can clear liver fire, nourish the heart, and moisten the lungs.

Mung beans: The cold and cooling nature of the mung bean can alleviate dryness in the body and dispel heat and toxins, and has the function of inhibiting the growth of bacteria.

Spinach: It nourishes *yin* and blood for people with *qi* and blood deficiency and with fire hyperactivity due to *yin* deficiency.

Green pepper: It can nourish the liver meridian, and is effective at cleansing the liver and brightening the eyes.

In addition, people with hyperactive liver fire should eat more fruit and vegetables rich in vitamins, drink more water, cut down on sweet and sour drinks, and eat less spicy and fried food. Purple cabbage, cauliflower, hawthorn, apples, and grapes are rich in minerals and have high calcium, magnesium, and silicon content. They have the effect of calming the mind and reducing internal heat.

Healthy and Delicious Recipes
Celery with Cashew Nuts
Ingredients: 200 g celery, 50 g cashew nuts, soy sauce and salt to taste

Method: ❶ Wash the celery, and cut into smaller chunks. ❷ Add some oil to the pan, pour in the celery chunks and stir

fry. Add salt to taste. When
the celery is cooked, add the
cashew nuts, and stir fry a few
times.

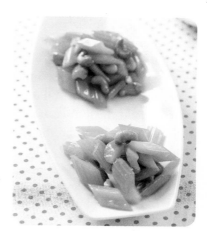

Effects: Celery is a food
that has a strong effect on
lowering blood pressure and
softening blood vessels. It
can help the liver to detoxify.
It also contains calcium and
potassium, which is very
beneficial to the body.

Mung Bean Buckwheat Paste

Ingredients: 70 g buckwheat,
50 g mung beans

Method: ❶ Wash the
mung beans and soak for ten
hours. ❷ Wash the buckwheat
and soak for three hours.
❸ Pour both the buckwheat
and mung beans into the
soybean machine. Add an
appropriate amount of water.
Mix until it becomes a paste.
(In the absence of a soybean

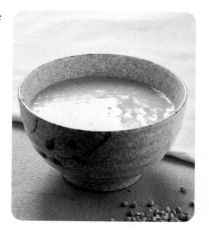

machine that has a cooking function, steam the buckwheat and
mung beans beforehand.)

Effects: Mung beans can clear heat and detoxify, while
buckwheat can soften blood vessels; both are effective at clearing
the liver and eyes. According to TCM theory, the heat clearing
function of mung beans lies in their skin, and the detoxification
function lies in their flesh. This recipe is for detoxification,
whereas mung bean soup boiled at a high heat is for dissipating
heat.

Stir Fried Indian Lettuce with Garlic

Ingredients: 300 g Indian lettuce, garlic, salt

Method: ❶ Wash the vegetables. Tear into sections by hand. ❷ Smash the garlic and mince it. ❸ Heat some oil in the pan. Add the lettuce and garlic, stir fry. ❹ When the lettuce is emerald green, add salt to taste.

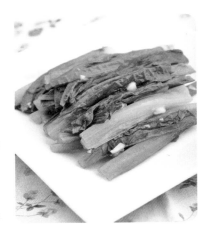

Effects: Indian lettuce clears the liver and invigorates the gallbladder. It can improve liver function, and help with liver detoxification. It can also stimulate the secretion of digestive juice and increase the appetite.

Broccoli with Cauliflower

Ingredients: 200 g each of broccoli and cauliflower, 100 g carrots, sugar, vinegar, sesame oil and salt to taste

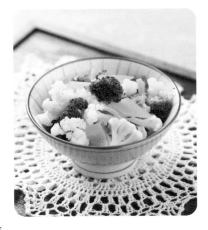

Method: ❶ Wash the broccoli and cauliflower separately. Break into smaller pieces. Wash, peel, and slice the carrots. ❷ Blanch all the vegetables, drain, and leave to cool. ❸ Place all the vegetables on a plate. Add sugar, vinegar, sesame oil, and salt to taste. Mix evenly.

Effects: Eating broccoli and cauliflower frequently can enhance the detoxification ability of the liver, improve the immunity of the body, and prevent colds and scurvy.

Dried Tangerine Peel & Kelp Porridge

Ingredients: 50 g each of kelp and round grain rice, dried tangerine peel, sugar

Method: ❶ Wash the dried tangerine peel. Wash the kelp, soak for two hours and mince. ❷ Wash the rice, and boil it in a pot with enough water. ❸ Add dried tangerine peel and minced kelp. Mix continuously. Continue cooking over a low heat until the porridge is almost done, and add sugar to taste.

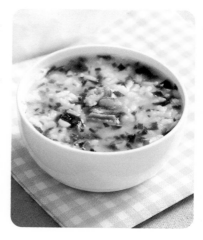

Effects: Regular consumption of dried tangerine peel & kelp porridge can dispel toxins in the body, relieve pressure on the liver for detoxification, replenish *qi* and nourish blood, clear heat, induce diuresis, as well as soothing the mind and keeping the body fit.

Bitter Gourd Salad

Ingredients: 100 g bitter gourd, sesame oil, salt

Method: ❶ Wash the bitter gourd and slice it. Blanch in hot water. ❷ Put the bitter gourd slices into cold water for a few minutes. Remove. ❸ Add sesame oil and salt, mix evenly.

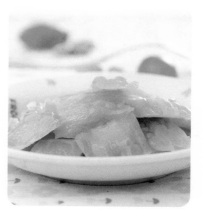

Effects: Bitter gourd clears heat, detoxifies, quenches thirst, and improves the mood. It is one of the best foods for reducing internal heat. Bitter gourd prepared this way is able to retain its medicinal effects, and is

also able to maintain its crisp taste to the maximum extent. This dish is ideal when you have rising heat in your body or when your appetite is low.

Hawthorn Rock Sugar Tea

Ingredients: 30 g hawthorns, 5 g green tea, rock sugar

Method: ❶ Wash and slice the hawthorns. Smash rock sugar into smaller pieces. ❷ Add water to a clay pot. Put in the hawthorn slices. ❸ Decoct it for ten minutes. Add the green tea leaves, followed by rock sugar.

Effects: Hawthorn is good for lowering blood pressure and reducing fats, invigorating the spleen and improving appetite, enhancing digestion and eliminating stagnation, promoting blood circulation and removing blood stasis. It can discharge blood stasis and toxins in the body and purify the blood. People who do not like sour flavors can add more rock sugar. Rinse your mouth after drinking to avoid damaging your teeth.

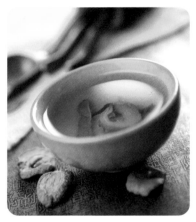

Water Spinach Salad

Ingredients: 250 g water spinach, garlic, sesame oil, salt

Method: ❶ Mince garlic. Wash the water spinach and cut into smaller lengths. ❷ Blanch the vegetable for two minutes, remove from water. ❸ Mix garlic mince and salt

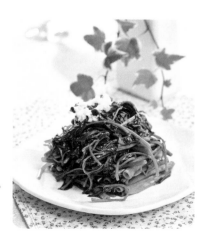

with a little water, add sesame oil and mix to a sauce. ❹ Pour the sauce over the water spinach, mix evenly.

Effects: Water spinach is sweet in flavor and cold in properties. It enters meridians of the liver, heart, large intestine, and small intestine. It clears heat and cools blood, and encourages diuresis while removing dampness. Water spinach can discharge the dampness toxins from the body.

Braised Beef Brisket with Tomato

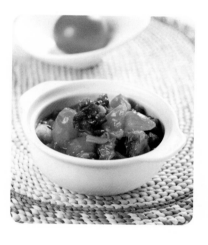

Ingredients: 250 g beef brisket, two tomatoes, one onion, salt

Method: ❶ Cut the beef brisket into smaller pieces. Blanch the meat, remove and leave it for later use. Wash the tomatoes and onion separately. Cut. Put them together in a stew pot. ❷ Add water and boil over a high heat. Add beef brisket. Lower the heat and continue stewing for 90 minutes. Add salt, increase to a high heat, and cook for another ten minutes.

Effects: The tomato has a cooling and slightly cold nature. It clears heat and quenches thirst, nourishing *yin* and cooling blood, as well as delaying aging.

Fried Shrimps with Chives

Ingredients: 200 g chives, 50 g shrimps, cooking wine, stock, scallions, ginger, garlic, sesame oil, salt

Method: ❶ Wash the shrimps. Devein them. Wash the chives and cut into smaller sections. Shred the scallions, ginger, garlic. ❷ Heat some oil in a pan, fry the scallions, ginger, and garlic shreds. Add the shrimps and stir fry. ❸ Add cooking wine, stock and salt, stir fry a little more. Add the chives and stir fry over a high heat. Add sesame oil.

Effects: Chives are warm in properties, and have the effects of tonifying the kidneys and *yang*, eliminating *yin*, and dispersing cold. It can strengthen the spleen and stomach *qi*, and is beneficial to liver detoxification.

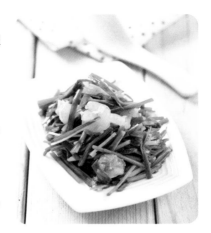

Chinese Yam Wolfberry Soybean Milk

Ingredients: 120 g Chinese yam, 40 g soybeans, 10 g wolfberries

Method: ❶ Peel yam, wash and cut into small pieces. ❷ Wash the soybeans and soak for ten hours until they are soft. Wash the wolfberries and soak them until they are soft. ❸ Place all the ingredients into the soybean machine, add some water and extract the juice. Garnish with a few wolfberries. (If the soybean machine does not have a cooking function, steam the Chinese yam and the soybeans beforehand.)

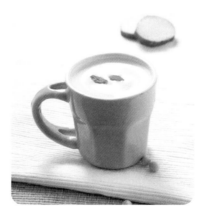

Effects: Chinese yam strengthens the spleen and tonifies deficiencies of the liver and kidneys, as well as soothing the mind.

Sweet Mustard Greens with Mushrooms

Ingredients: six mushrooms, 250 g sweet mustard greens, salt

Method: ❶ Wash the sweet mustard greens, cut; separate

the leaf stalks from the leaves. ❷ Wash the mushrooms, soak them in warm water and remove the stems. Cut into pieces. ❸ Heat some oil in a pan, throw in the mustard greens stalks, stir fry until about 60% cooked, add salt followed by the leaves, continue stir frying. ❹ Add the mushroom pieces and the warm water used to soak the mushrooms. Cook until the stalks of the mustard greens are soft.

Effects: Sweet mustard greens have a cooling properties, and enter the liver, spleen, and lung meridians. They can remove stagnation, invigorate blood circulation, detoxify, break up stagnated *qi*, and reduce swelling. The components in mustard greens can encourage blood circulation and enhance the liver's detoxification function.

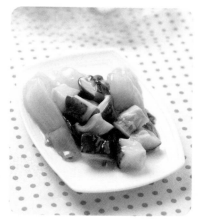

Lettuce in Milk Sauce

Ingredients: 200 g lettuce, 100 g broccoli, 125 g fresh milk, starch, stock, salt

Method: ❶ Wash the lettuce and cut it up. Wash the broccoli and break it into smaller florets. ❷ Heat the oil in a pan. Add lettuce and broccoli, and stir fry. ❸ Add salt and stock to taste. Dish onto a plate. ❹ Boil milk, and add stock and starch to make thick sauce. Pour over the vegetables.

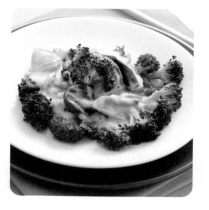

Effects: Lettuce clears the liver and gall bladder, which helps detoxification.

Pomegranate Juice with Honey

Ingredients: one pomegranate, honey

    Method: ❶ Wash the pomegranate. Remove the skin and extract the seeds. ❷ Put the pomegranate seeds in a juicer, add an appropriate amount of water, and turn on the juicer. ❸ Strain the juice. Add honey to taste.

    Effects: Pomegranate can clear heat and detoxify, nourish the blood and invigorate blood circulation, as well as relieve diarrhea; therefore, it is ideal for patients with chronic diarrhea and women with prolonged menstrual periods. Women doing a beauty detox and maintaining healthy skin should add a little pomegranate skin when making the juice as an added benefit.

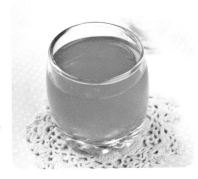

Carrot and Orange Juice

Ingredients: two oranges, one carrot

    Method: ❶ Wash the oranges, remove the skin, and break into segments. ❷ Wash, peel, and cut the carrot into pieces. ❸ Place the orange segments and carrot pieces into the juicer. Juice them.

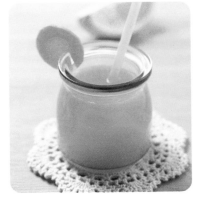

    Effects: Oranges taste sweet and sour. They can stimulate the stomach to enhance the appetite, relax the diaphragm, and strengthen the spleen. People who socialize often and like to drink should consume some orange juice before or after meals to reduce the burden on the liver in detoxification.

5. Tea Therapy to Detoxify the Liver

While we are at work, our eyes are on our computers and mobile phone screens. When we get home at night, we watch TV. Before going to bed, we spend a little time reading e-books. After a while, we begin to feel dizzy and experience eye pain. Our bodies are sending us a signal telling us that our livers need to detoxify and our eyes need to rest. During your rest time, make a cup of tea. This can clear your liver and brighten your eyes.

Chrysanthemum Tea

Ingredients: ten chrysanthemum buds

Method: ❶ Put the chrysanthemum buds into a teapot. Pour in boiling water. ❷ Soak for 3 to 5 minutes.

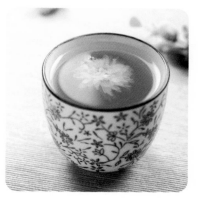

Effects: Chrysanthemum can disperse wind-heat, relieve heat, and generate saliva. Regular consumption can moisten the throat and brighten the eyes. It is a very good eye-wellness tea for office workers.

Chrysanthemum and Cassia Seed Tea

Ingredients: five chrysanthemum buds, eight wolfberries, cassia seeds

Method: ❶ Put the chrysanthemum buds, wolfberries, and cassia seeds into a cup. Pour in boiling water. ❷ Soak for five minutes.

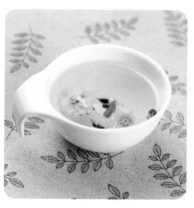

Effects: Chrysanthemum buds and wolfberries are both

effective at expelling liver toxins and protecting the eyes. When the two are combined, they create an even stronger effect in nourishing the liver and brightening the eyes.

Bitter Gourd Mint Tea

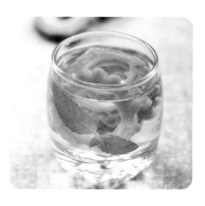

Ingredients: three mint leaves and three slices of bitter gourd, rock sugar

Method: ❶ Put the mint leaves, bitter gourd slices, and rock sugar into a cup. Pour in boiling water. ❷ Cover and let it sit for five minutes before drinking.

Effects: Mint leaves are effective at expelling gastrointestinal toxins, reducing dampness swelling, moving the bowels, and promoting weight loss. They also have the effect of dispelling pathogenic wind for improving eyesight, dissipating heat, and relieving itching. They can also relieve headaches, dizziness, sore throat and hoarseness, and skin irritation. The active protein in bitter gourd can improve the immune system and enhance antiviral function. Moreover, bitter gourd can accelerate the excretion of toxins in the body. In hot weather, drinking some bitter gourd and mint tea can refresh the mind, clear heat and detoxify, lower the heart fire, and eliminate heart toxins.

Honeysuckle Tea

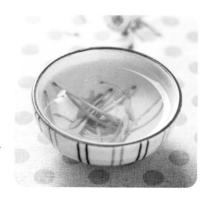

Ingredients: 15 to 20 honeysuckle flowers

Method: ❶ Put the honeysuckle flowers into a cup. Add boiling water. ❷ Drink when it has cooled.

Effects: Honeysuckle has a good detoxification effect, and works as a bactericide and anti-inflammatory cure for influenza, periodontitis, and tonsillitis. Drinking it can enhance your immunity to the influenza virus during flu season.

Honeysuckle and Mung Bean Tea

Ingredients: 30 honeysuckle flowers, mung beans

Method: ❶ Wash the honeysuckle and mung beans separately. Put in a pot, add water and bring to the boil over a high heat. ❷ Turn off the heat after ten minutes. Let it cool slightly before drinking.

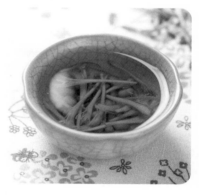

Effects: Mung beans are well known for their ability to break down toxins and expel them. When boiled over a high heat, mung bean soup is very effective at relieving heat. Add some honeysuckle flowers to it and it becomes a very practical drink in summer for relieving heat and generating bodily fluids.

Cassia Seeds Tea

Ingredients: cassia seeds, green tea

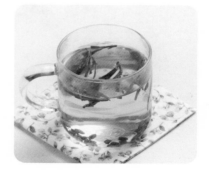

Method: ❶ Put the cassia seeds and green tea into a cup. Add boiling water. ❷ Soak for ten minutes.

Effects: Cassia seeds can clear the liver and brighten the eyes, and can eliminate liver toxins. When people with ascending hyperactive liver *yang* have symptoms such as headaches, dizziness, and insomnia, they can use pillows stuffed with cassia seeds as an effective adjuvant therapy.

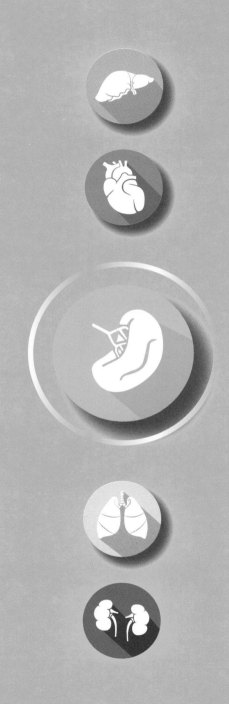

Chapter Four
Detoxifying the Spleen

A mong the five *zang* organs, the spleen is associated to the earth element. The earth is the mother of all things, with the trait of being reliable. It is the point where life begins, and also the point where life ends. The spleen can transform *qi* and blood. It provides nourishment to all parts of the body, and is required for the continuation of life. The spleen loves warmth and dryness, and hates cold and dampness. If you eat without restraint, and do not limit your consumption of cold and cooling foods, you will harm your internal organs. Therefore, if you nourish your spleen and stomach, your *qi* and blood will be abundant, and your *yang qi* will regulate its ascent and descent without creating any problems.

According to TCM, the spleen governs transportation and transformation. Transportation includes distribution, while transformation refers to a change. During the fetal period, we rely solely on maternal nutrition for survival. After birth, with the gradual maturity of the organs responsible for digestion, our nutritional needs come from the food that goes into our bodies. The food we consume is not directly absorbed and utilized. Instead, it needs to undergo a series of physiological metabolizations, such as decomposition and transformation, through organs such as the spleen and stomach, to regenerate *qi* and blood and bodily fluids, and to nourish the viscera, meridians, limbs, and bones. In the case of a malfunction of the spleen and stomach, various ailments can develop such as digestive and absorption disorders, malnutrition, deficiency of *qi* and blood, deficiency of meridians, and muscle atrophy.

There are two substances in the body that need to be

transported and transformed by the spleen and stomach. First is the essence of water and grains, i.e., foods that modern nutritional studies consider as containing components such as carbohydrates, fats, protein, minerals, and vitamins. Second is fluid, which is regarded as the most important transportation carrier and biochemical reaction medium in metabolism.

If a person wants to live healthily, they must first constantly ingest food and convert it into the various nutrients required for life functions. However, food alone is not enough. What you eat must be converted to *qi*, blood, and bodily fluids that can be absorbed and are needed by the body (TCM refers all normal fluids in the body, except for blood, as bodily fluids, which mainly come from the water and grains consumed). *Qi*, blood, and bodily fluids are the three basic substances that constitute and maintain life functions. None of the body's five *zang* organs, six *fu* organs, meridians, muscles, bones, and skin can be separated from the warmth, moisture, and nutrition of *qi*, blood, and bodily fluids. Only when the *qi* and blood are vigorous, the bodily fluids are abundant, the *zang-fu* organs are nourished, and the meridians are unobstructed, can mental activities be calm. Living a long and healthy life is then achievable.

After fluid is generated from what we eat and drink, some of it is absorbed and transported by the spleen and stomach. This is then distributed to the other parts of the body to perform its role in moistening, lubricating and nourishing. The rest is transformed into sweat and urine through gasification that takes place in the lungs and kidneys, and is discharged from the body. When there is an abnormality in the function of the spleen's transportation and transformation of fluid, the dispersion and excretion of fluid will not be able to be carried out, and it will stay stagnant in the body, causing pathological dampness, phlegm, fluid retention, and edema, leading to many ailments. Illnesses caused by exogenous dampness pathogen can also harm the spleen and stomach. Therefore, for most diseases related to water-dampness in the body, TCM will use treatment methods that can invigorate and strengthen the spleen, especially those that can invigorate the spleen *yang*[1] and tonify the spleen *qi*[2] to dispel water and encourage diuresis.

1. Are There Toxins in Your Spleen?

Most of the issues are caused by inappropriate diet and excessive drinking. Common symptoms include abdominal distension, stomach distension, and loose stools. Once the spleen and stomach are damaged, therapy treatment will take a long time. The following symptoms show that your spleen has been "poisoned."

A smooth, white tongue coating with teeth marks: The tongue coating can reflect a person's physical condition. If the tongue coating is white, feels greasy, and has teeth marks on the edge, it may be an indication of spleen deficiency. According to TCM theory, when this happens, the transportation and transformation of fluid and dampness will be obstructed, causing stagnating dampness on the tongue, as well as hypertrophy of the tongue body. When the swollen tongue edge presses against the teeth, imprints will form. You are advised to eat less food that has a cold nature and cooling effect to avoid stimulating the spleen and stomach. Eat more vegetarian food and less meat to gradually regulate the condition of your stomach and intestines.

Edema: The main symptom of spleen deficiency is systemic edema, with thigh and calf edema being the most serious. When you press it, it will sag and not rebound easily. This is a result of an

---

[1] The *yang qi* of the spleen, as opposed to the *yin* of the spleen, is the warm driving force and the ascending clear side of the spleen.

[2] The essential *qi* of the spleen is manifested through its transportation and transformation functions, the ascending of clear matter, and the control of blood. Spleen *qi* also refers to the material basis of the physiological function of the spleen.

inappropriate diet, often eating spicy and stimulating food, feeling depressed, thinking or worrying too much, and dysfunctional work and rest. Damage to the spleen affects the proper functioning of the transportation and transformation of fluid-dampness, which will lead to water retention and edema. Pregnant women belong to a special group of people; most of them will also experience edema in the second trimester of their pregnancy. One type is due to the enlarged uterus compressing the legs, which affects the flow of returning blood, leading to more serious edema in the lower limbs. If this happens to you, eat a lighter diet and engage in proper exercise to reduce edema. The other type is generalized edema, known as pregnancy edema in medical science. After seven weeks of pregnancy, if your body weight increases too quickly each week, seek medical treatment immediately.

Excessive leukorrhea: The spleen is in charge of the body's discharge of moisture. If the amount of moisture exceeds the absorption range of the spleen, there will be excess moisture retained in the body. An increase in leukorrhea is one indication of this situation.

Pale lips and pimples around the mouth: The area around the lips is closely related to the spleen. When the toxins in the spleen are not discharged from the body and accumulate, they will burst out through these places. Because the spleen has such a close relationship with the mouth, the color of the lips is an indicator of the situation of *qi* and blood. When there is a dysfunction of the spleen's transportation ability[1], the *qi* and blood will be insufficient. The lips and tongue will be pale, even yellow, and pimples will emerge around the lips. Include some food that could tonify spleen-*qi* in your daily diet, such as lotus seeds and roots, Chinese yam, French beans, cowpeas, carrots, potatoes, onions, and oyster mushrooms.

---

[1] Pathological changes caused by abnormal spleen function in transportation and transformation.

Pigmentation on the face: Most facial pigmentation is caused by endocrine disorders, which can be regulated through TCM treatment but rarely permanently cured. High mental pressure, emotional disorders, neurological disorders, and physical fatigue can also cause pigmentation. According to TCM theory, pigmentation is blood stasis. Discolored spots or patches on the face are often related to *qi* stagnation and blood stasis. With spleen deficiency, the disrupted circulation of *qi* and blood means that blood cannot be pushed forward, causing stasis that gives rise to discolored spots on the face. Syndrome differentiation treatment is required in addition to developing good living habits and maintaining an optimistic mood.

Yellowish complexion: A yellowish complexion is a sign of insufficient *qi* and bodily fluids in the spleen, which is not able to provide enough nutrition to the body. Some people's faces looked withered and yellow, and others are yellow and swollen. People with a weak stomach and a spleen deficiency should avoid spicy, irritating, raw, and cold food. They should eat regular meals at set hours and portions, chewing well and swallow slowly.

2. Habits That Harm the Spleen

The spleen must be protected well because if it is damaged, the body's ability to defend itself and produce antibodies will decline. To protect the spleen, we must first change the following habits.

Overeating: Overeating will result in a large amount of food accumulating and stagnating in the digestive tract. This makes it difficult for the transportation and transformation function of the spleen and stomach to work, and also hinders the operation of the *qi*, resulting in abdominal distension, decreased appetite, nausea, and vomiting. It has always been regarded as the standard by wellness dietitians through the ages to eat a moderate diet and not to eat until the stomach is full. Overeating is usually accompanied by chewing and swallowing too fast. The adverse effects of this kind of eating will begin to manifest when one reaches middle age. When the spleen declines, health will decline. Therefore, overeating is a very harmful habit.

Sitting for a long time: TCM stresses that wellness and healthcare should focus on balance, and nothing should be excessive. Overusing the eyes hurts the blood, lying down for prolonged period hurts *qi*, sitting for a long time hurts the muscles, standing for a long time hurts the bones, and walking for a long time hurts the tendons. TCM refers to this protracted accumulation of injuries as *wu lao*—the five injury factors, of which the most closely related to the spleen is the injury caused by sitting for a long time. The spleen and stomach, being the source of transformation of *qi* and blood, work to nourish the muscles. Therefore, only when the spleen and stomach are healthy and the *qi* and blood are abundant can the muscles be strong and powerful. Sitting for a long time will cause the muscles to be slack and weak, seriously diminishing energy consumption, leading to energy surplus and deposition, and in turn burdening the spleen. Therefore, we should exercise often, using equipment appropriately and also including some workouts to strengthen the muscles. Take regular walks and do more exercise that encourage oxygen intake to strengthen the spleen and stomach.

Regular consumption of raw and cold food: The spleen and stomach are digestive organs, or food processing factories. The spleen in TCM includes the functions of digestion, absorption, and energy metabolism of Western medicine. People with a spleen deficiency always feel weak during the digestion process, and suffer cold in the stomach, because the stomach and intestines have used up their energy in the digestion of raw and cold food. According to TCM theory, food is differentiated into cold, hot, warm, or cooling natural characteristics. Consuming food that is too cold will cause major damage to the spleen and stomach. These four natural attributes are TCM's induction and summary of foods' reaction to the human body. For example, TCM regards crab as having a very cold nature. When steaming crabs, add perilla leaves. When eating crabs, use a ginger juice dip. Add a little mustard to the sauce, and drink an appropriate amount of yellow rice wine afterwards. The purpose is to remove the cold in the food and protect the *yang* in the spleen and stomach. It is advisable for people with a spleen deficiency to eat sweet and warm food often, such as glutinous rice, black rice, sorghum, millet, oats, pumpkin, lentils, red dates, longan, walnuts, and chestnuts.

Living in cold and humid places: The main characteristic of the spleen is that it likes dryness and hates dampness. Because the spleen belongs to the earth element, it very much needs the warmth, transpiration, and gasification of *yang qi* to transform *qi* and blood and transport bodily fluids. Therefore, in our daily life, we must avoid moist and damp places. Once the damp level in the room rises, we must ventilate it to reduce the indoor humidity.

3. Massage Therapy to Detoxify the Spleen

The main function of the spleen is to transport and transform. It converts the essence of nutrients into *qi*, blood and bodily fluids, and then transports it to the various viscera and tissues of the body through the heart and lungs, so as to meet the needs to life functions. As a result, spleen deficiency syndrome is more common than excess syndrome. Even cases of the latter usually involve some degree of deficiency. For example, in cases where there is food retention and dampness obstruction[1], spleen deficiency will develop over time. TCM attaches great importance to the regulation of spleen and stomach functions. One of the methods is massage therapy. Using press-knead

---

[1] Dampness pathogens block the middle *jiao* (the spleen and stomach), weakening transportation and transformation functions. The main clinical features are fullness of the epigastrium and heaviness of the limbs.

manipulation on the spleen meridian can enhance the organ's transportation and transformation function.

Massage the Daimai Acupoint

Many people are puzzled as to why they still gain weight when they eat so little. Although we know that losing weight does not happen overnight, despite the effort we put in, we are not always successful. Nowadays, remaining sedentary is very common, and this can hurt the spleen, causing disruption to its transformation and transportation function. Abdominal fat, which is very common now, is the result of the malfunctioning of the spleen.

This brings us to the remarkable Daimai acupoints, located on the Dai Meridian, which is one of the eight extra meridians. It is a horizontal meridian, and circles the waist. Massaging the Daimai acupoints can speed up *qi* and blood circulation, and can alleviate cold and pain in the lower back as well as dysmenorrhea. Apply press-knead manipulation on these points to strengthen spleen *yang*, invigorate *yang qi*, and dissipate the accumulated fluid, phlegm, and dampness in the abdomen. Massaging the Daimai acupoints can also enhance intestinal peristalsis and encourage defecation.

Acupoint location: On both sides of the abdomen, at the intersection of the vertical line at the free end of the 11th rib and the horizontal line of the umbilicus. Or, draw a horizontal line with the navel as the center, and then draw a vertical line with the front end of the armpit as the starting point. The intersection

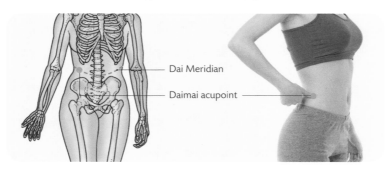

Dai Meridian

Daimai acupoint

of the two lines is the Daimai acupoint.

Massage method: Women with irregular menstruation and abnormal leukorrhea can hit the Daimai acupoints 100 times with their clenched fist when they get up every morning. For abdominal obesity, use the thenar of the palm (the raised part at the root of the thumb) to knead the entire Dai Meridian twice a day, for 5 to 10 minutes each time, and then apply pressure to the painful part on the meridian. If you persist, abdominal obesity will gradually reduce.

Press-Knead the Taibai Acupoint

The Taibai acupoints are responsible for supporting the spleen meridian. When pressing Taibai acupoints, take note whether there is any numbness or swelling pain that would indicate issues with the spleen.

Acupoint location: In the metatarsal region of both feet, in the depression at the proximal end of the first metatarsophalangeal (big toe) joint where the red and white skin meet.

Massage method: Press-knead the Taibai acupoints in a clockwise or anticlockwise direction repeatedly, for three minutes each time.

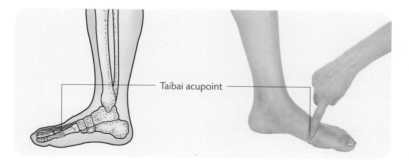

Taibai acupoint

Massage the Xuehai Acupoint

The Xuehai acupoint belongs to the spleen meridian. Since the spleen generates and governs the blood, its first function is to regulate blood and treat various blood-related ailments. The

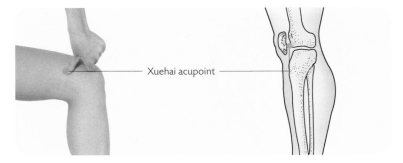

Xuehai acupoint

second function is to nourish the blood and dispel wind, as well as treating skin allergies and itching. The third function is to maintain beauty, especially for women, who are blood-based. When there is blood deficiency, the skin is not able to restore its beauty, therefore allowing pigmentation, wrinkles, and roughness to develop.

Acupoint location: On both legs. To locate it, flex your knee. It is on the inner side of the thigh, 2 cun above the medial end of the patella base, at the bulge of the medial portion of the quadriceps femoris.

Massage method: Knead-press the Xuehai acupoints in a clockwise or anticlockwise direction repeatedly, for three minutes each time.

4. Diet Therapy to Detoxify the Spleen

Qi and blood, bodily fluids, and essence are generated in the spleen and stomach. For the *zang-fu* (viscera) to function with vigor, the spleen and stomach have to be strong. The spleen and stomach are also the hub of *qi* movement[1]. The coordination of the spleen and stomach encourages and regulates the body's metabolic function and ensures the coordination and balance of life functions.

---

[1] The movement of *qi* takes the basic forms of ascending, descending, exiting and entering.

Sweet Food

Have you noticed that when you eat rice, rice porridge, or corn, you perceive a slightly sweet flavor in your mouth? Some warm and tonic ingredients, such as ginseng, longan, red dates, and Chinese yam, do taste sweet. As a matter of fact, all grains are produced from the soil, and are categorized as sweet foods. These foods have the best effect in nourishing the spleen and stomach. Among the *zang-fu*, the functions of the spleen are transportation and transformation. It breaks down the food that enters our body, and transform it into nutrient essence. The nutrients digested and absorbed by the body and then the spleen will transport this essence to the whole body. Sweet foods can relieve contracture[2], moisten dryness, nourish, and tonify the spleen, enhancing its transportation and transformation functions.

Sweet flavor can relieve muscle tension. When the spleen function is healthy, the body will look full with a rosy complexion. Because the sweet flavor is ascribed to the spleen and stomach, it can improve their functions and supplement their deficiencies, while indirectly tonifying and nourishing other viscera. For people who are physically weak and suffer from insufficient *qi* and blood, including more sweet foods in their diet can gradually improve their physique and strengthen their body.

Ginseng: With its sweet and slight bitter flavor, ginseng is good for invigorating *qi* to relieve desertion[3], strengthening the spleen and lungs, calming the heart, and sharpening the mind, as well as nourishing blood and bodily fluids.

Longan: Rich in glucose, sucrose, protein, various vitamins, and trace elements, longans can be used to treat physical weakness or mental decline after illness thanks to their nourishing effect.

Chinese yam: Effective at enhancing the digestion and absorption function of the spleen and stomach, Chinese yam is

---

[2] Relieving spasms and convulsions caused by the wind-cold.
[3] The treatment of *qi* desertion through medicines that tonify vital energy.

used as a medicine as well as a food, and can evenly reinforce[1] the spleen and stomach. It is suitable for consumption for both spleen *yang* deficiency and stomach *yin* deficiency.

However, excessive consumption of sweet flavors will cause an imbalance of kidney *qi*. It will fail to nourish the body, and will cause the face to darken, bringing bone pain and hair loss. Therefore, sweet foods should be eaten in moderation.

Yellow Food

Yellow in the five elements represents the color of the earth, and in the five *zang* organs the spleen is associated with the earth. Therefore, according to TCM theory, yellow corresponds to the spleen and the earth. Therefore, when yellow food is taken into the body, it mainly acts on the spleen and stomach. Yellow foods such as millet, corn, pumpkin, and soybeans are good for strengthening the spleen and stomach.

Millet: It is good for people with deficiency and heat in the spleen and stomach, and for those who eat only a little but feel full and bloated. Millet is effective at regulating the middle warmer (spleen and stomach) and is good for the kidneys as well.

Corn: It can invigorate the spleen and dispel dampness, regulate the middle warmer and stimulate the appetite. It is good for the kidneys, and it also stimulates the intellectual side of the heart (the mind).

Pumpkin: It has a beneficial effect for the stomach, and is rich in carbohydrates and pectin, which can protect the gastric mucosa.

Modern research has found that yellow food is rich in the B vitamins, vitamin D, and β-carotene. From the nutritional perspective, vitamins do not contain energy, but bodily processes such as digestion, absorption, and metabolism are driven by the

---

[1] The use of gentle tonic prescriptions to treat patients with chronic weak physique and diseases that develop slowly.

effects of vitamins.

In addition, some white food can strengthen the spleen when fried yellow. For example, in TCM, it is believed that barley has a better effect on the spleen when it is cooked. Therefore, in clinical practice, people with a spleen deficiency are often asked to fry barley until the grains turn slightly yellow, and eat them when they are cooked. When barley is used as medicine or food, it can strengthen the spleen and dispel dampness. People nowadays often eat big meals. When the intake of rich food is too much, obesity will develop and blood lipid levels will increase. Barley contains a lot of unsaturated fatty acids, which can dispel dampness and resolve phlegm, and also reduce cholesterol. It is especially suitable for people with a phlegm-dampness constitution.

Delicious Healthy Recipes
Seaweed-Wrapped Rice

Ingredients: 100 g glutinous rice, one egg, one piece of seaweed, ham, cucumber, salad dressing, rice vinegar

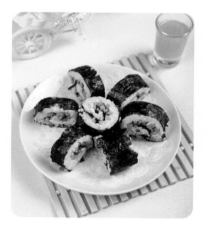

Method: ❶ Steam the glutinous rice. Add rice vinegar, and mix evenly. Leave to cool. ❷ Wash the cucumber. Cut into long strips, and add rice vinegar to marinade. Cut ham into strips. ❸ Heat the oil in a pan. Pour in the beaten egg into the pan, and spread it like a pancake. Cut into thin strips. Lay the glutinous rice on the seaweed. Lay the cucumber, ham, and egg strips evenly on the rice. ❹ Spread some salad dressing, roll it up and cut the roll into pieces of about 2 cm in length.

Effects: Glutinous rice can warm the spleen and stomach, and nourish the middle qi[1] of the spleen and stomach. Regular consumption can nourish and strengthen the body.

Lily and Barley Paste

Ingredients: 50 g barley, 20 g dried lily bulb, sugar

Method: ❶ Soak the dried lily bulb and barley for three hours. Drain. Put them in a soybean machine, and add some water. ❷ Turn on the machine and make the mixture into a paste. Add sugar to taste. (If the soybean machine does not have a cooking function, steam the barley and dried lily bulb together.)

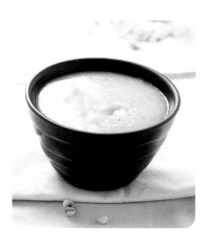

Effects: Barley strengthens the spleen and stomach, clearing away heat and moistening the lungs. Lily bulb invigorates the spleen-stomach and replenishes qi, clears heat and detoxifies. When these two are combined, they can clear and moisten the lungs, and discharge the dampness toxin from body.

Lotus Root Salad

Ingredients: 250 g lotus root, scallions, ginger, garlic, white vinegar, salt

Method: ❶ Cut the scallions into tiny pieces, shred ginger, and slice garlic. ❷ Wash the lotus root, peel, and slice. ❸ Blanch the lotus root slices, dish out. Add scallions, ginger shreds, garlic slices, vinegar, and salt. Mix evenly.

---

[1] Also known as the qi of the spleen and stomach. The spleen, stomach, and small intestine's physiological functions such as digestion, absorption, transportation, and elevating clear qi to lower turbid qi.

Effects: Lotus root has high nutritional value, but its value is different when it is raw and when it is cooked. Raw lotus root eliminates blood stasis and cools the blood, clearing heat and uplifting the spirit. Cooked lotus root can strengthen the spleen and *qi*, nourish the heart, and tonify the blood. Therefore, cooked lotus root is suitable for people with weak spleen *qi*, while raw lotus root is suitable for people with hyperactive stomach heat.

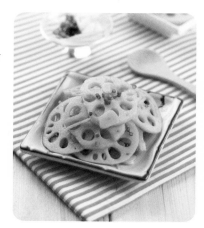

White Fungus and Peanut Soup

Ingredients: 15 g white fungus, 50 g peanuts, ten red dates, sugar

Method: ❶ Soak white fungus in warm water, wash. Remove the pits of the red dates, wash. ❷ Boil water in a pot, add peanuts, red dates and white fungus. ❸ When the peanuts are soft and cooked, add sugar to taste.

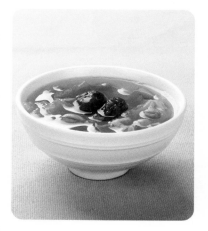

Effects: Peanuts can help the spleen to detoxify, but they are not easy to digest. They can be eaten cooked or stewed.

Braised Baby Cabbage with Shii-take

Ingredients: 300 g baby cabbage, 30 g shii-take, garlic, sugar, salt

Method: ❶ Wash the baby cabbage. Remove the root.

Mince garlic. ❷ Wash the shii-take, remove the stems, and cut into slices. ❸ Heat some oil in the pan, and fry the minced garlic and shii-take slices until fragrant. Add the baby cabbage and stir fry. Lower the heat, and add some water to braise it. Then add salt and sugar to taste.

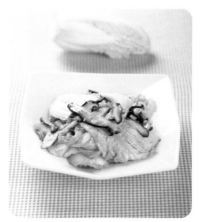

Effects: In addition to the nutrients that most mushrooms have, shii-take also contain lentinan, which can inhibit tumors and reduce blood lipids.

Chinese Yam Lentil Cake

Ingredients: Chinese yam 250 g, lentil 50 g, shredded red dates, shredded bell pepper, starch

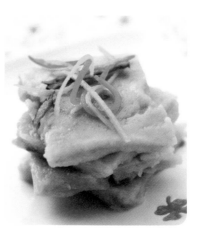

Method: ❶ Wash the yam, peel, and slice thinly. Cook the yam and lentils separately. Mash them when they have cooled down. Add starch and

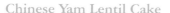

water and mix into a paste. Place the paste in a bowl. ❷ Put the bowl into a steamer and steam for 25 to 30 minutes over a high heat. When it has cooled down, cut it into smaller pieces. Garnish with shredded red dates and shredded bell pepper.

Effects: People with a poor appetite should eat more yams to strengthen their spleen and dissipate dampness.

Ginseng Lotus Seed Porridge

Ingredients: 10 g ginseng, ten lotus seeds, 50 g round grain

rice, black sesame seeds, rock sugar

Method: ❶ Soak the ginseng in water until it softens. Slice. ❷ Remove the plumule in the lotus seeds. Wash and soak them for three hours. ❸ Wash the rice. Put the rice, ginseng, and lotus seeds in a pot. Add water and boil. When the porridge is cooked, add rock sugar and black sesame seeds. Mix evenly.

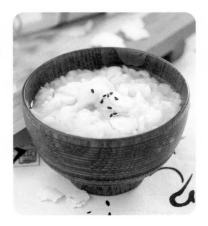

Effects: This porridge invigorates vital energy and sharpens the mind. In addition to helping the spleen to detoxify, it also encourages children's intellectual development. Ginseng, however, is a tonic and too much should not be eaten.

Mashed Potato with Apple

Ingredients: one apple, one potato, walnuts

Method: ❶ Wash the potato. Steam, and remove the skin. Cut into smaller pieces. ❷ Wash the apple, remove its core, and cut it into smaller pieces. ❸ Put the potato and apple into a soybean machine. Add some water and blend to fine paste. (If the soybean machine does not have a cooking function, precook the potato.)

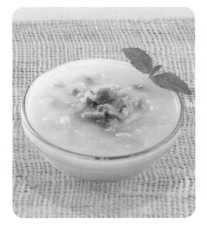

❹ Break the walnuts into tiny pieces, and sprinkle on the mashed potato and apple mixture.

Effects: Patients with a weak spleen and stomach, abdominal pain, and constipation should eat potatoes more often. This mashed potato dish is also rich in dietary fiber, which is an ideal food therapy for expelling spleen and intestinal toxins.

Oatmeal and Pumpkin Porridge

Ingredients: 30 g oats, 50 g round grain rice, half a pumpkin, scallions, salt

Method: ❶ Wash the rice and soak for half an hour.
❷ Wash the pumpkin, remove the skin, and cut into slices. Cut the scallions into tiny pieces, and leave aside. ❸ Put the rice in a pot, add water, and cook over a high heat. When it starts to boil, lower the heat and continue cooking for 20 minutes. Add pumpkin slices, and cook over a low heat for another ten minutes. Add oats, and cook for ten more minutes. Turn off the heat. Garnish with scallions and add salt to taste.

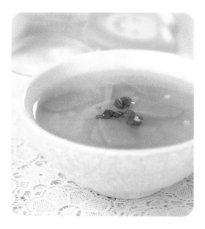

Effects: Pumpkin has a warm nature. It moistens the lungs and replenishes *qi*, beautifying the skin, strengthening the stomach and digestion, and enhancing the detoxification function of the spleen and stomach.

Corn and Egg Soup

Ingredients: 100 g corn kernels, two eggs, sugar, salt

Method: ❶ Whisk the eggs, and leave aside. ❷ Put the corn kernels into a pot, add water, and bring to the boil.

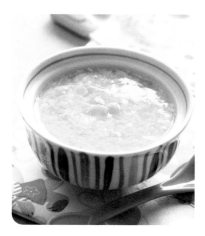

Lower the heat, and cook for another 20 minutes. ❸ Pour the beaten egg slowly into the pot, stirring all the time. Turn up the heat, and once it starts to boil, add sugar and salt to taste.

Effects: Corn is good for nourishing the lungs and calming the heart, moistening the intestines and relieving constipation. It can also help to expel toxins in the body and delay the aging process.

Millet and Red Date Porridge

Ingredients: 50 g millet, two red dates, honey

Method: ❶ Wash the millet and red dates separately. Put the red dates in a pot, add water, and bring to the boil. Add the millet only when the water is boiling. ❷ Cook over a high heat until it starts boiling. Lower the heat until the porridge is cooked. ❸ When the porridge has cooled down, add honey to taste.

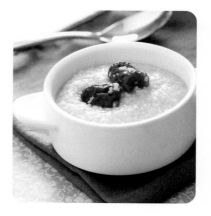

Effects: Millet and red dates are very good tonic foods for the blood, and are suitable for cooking into porridge. When the millet red date porridge is cooked, the substance that resembles oil paste floating on the surface is called "rice oil." This is very good for eliminating pathogenic cold toxins from the body.

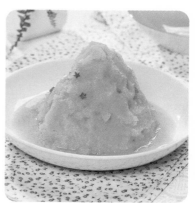

Stir Fried Sweet Potato Paste

Ingredients: two sweet potatoes, sugar

Method: ❶ Wash the

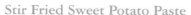

sweet potatoes and steam them. Peel off the skin while they are still hot. Mash them, and add sugar to taste. ❷ Heat some oil in a pan, move the pan to coat it with oil to prevent the sweet potato from sticking to it. ❸ Pour in the mashed sweet potato, and stir fry quickly until it changes color.

Effects: Sweet potato can warm and nourish the stomach. Eat some stir fried sweet potato paste in the cold winter season to help expel pathogenic cold toxins.

Mango Sago

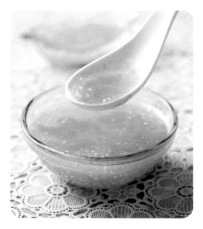

Ingredients: one mango, 200 ml milk, sago, honey

Method: ❶ Boil some water in a pot, and add sago when it starts to boil. Cook over a high heat for ten minutes. Turn off the heat and leave it covered for 15 minutes. Dish out and rinse in cold water. ❷ Change the water in the pot and bring it to the boil. Pour in the rinsed sago. Cook over a high heat for five minutes. Turn off the heat and leave it covered for 15 minutes. ❸ Wash and dice the mango. Mix the mango with honey, sago, and milk evenly.

Effects: This dish is a delicious summer dessert suitable for people with indigestion, fatigue, limb weakness, and toxin sedimentation.

Ginger and Orange Peel Dessert Drink

Ingredients: 10 g ginger, 10 g orange peel, brown sugar

Method: ❶ Shred the ginger and cut the orange peel into tiny pieces. ❷ Evenly mix the shredded ginger and orange peel with brown sugar. ❸ Add water and boil it to make into a dessert drink.

Effects: Ginger warms the stomach and dispels cold. Orange peel stimulates the appetite and enhances the smooth flow of *qi*. Combining the two can nurse the spleen and stomach back to health, improving the appetite, strengthening the spleen, and promoting digestion. Adding a little ginger to food of a cold nature can reduce the degree of "coldness," expel cold toxins, and protect the spleen and stomach.

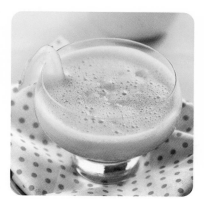

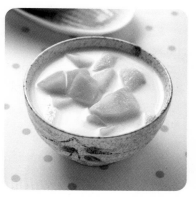

Papaya and Pear Milk

Ingredients: 250 g fresh milk, 100 g snow pear, 100 g papaya, honey

Method: ❶ Wash the snow pear and papaya separately. Peel the skin off them and remove the seeds. Cut into small pieces. ❷ Place them into a stew pot and add milk. Add water to the pot and bring to the boil. When the snow pear and papaya are soft, add some honey.

Effects: Papaya strengthens the stomach, encourages digestion, relaxes the muscles, and unblocks the collaterals. When combined with snow pear and honey, it can also moisten the lungs and alleviate coughing. It is a good detoxification drink in summer and autumn.

5. Tea Therapy to Detoxify the Spleen

It can take a long time to lose weight. The biggest problem is that the fat that we work so hard to shed piles back on quickly as soon as we relax our efforts even a little. Some people find it difficult to lose weight no matter what they do. Such situations are usually because the food taken into the stomach is not digested by the spleen, and is left to accumulate in the body. The following tea recipes strengthen the spleen, making weight loss simple and effective.

Lotus Leaf Tea

Ingredient: half of a dried lotus leaf

Method: ❶ Cut up the dried lotus leaf, put it in a teapot, and add boiling water. ❷ Leave it in the teapot for five minutes. Strain and drink.

Effects: Lotus leaf clears and relieves heat, dispels dampness and stasis, encourages diuresis and defecation, and can help to discharge the remaining toxins in the gastrointestinal tract. People who want to lose weight should drink lotus leaf tea often, because it can strengthen the spleen, invigorate *yang*, and reduce the absorption of fats in the body.

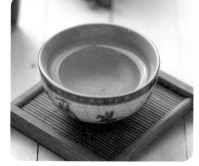

Lotus Leaf and Osmanthus Tea

Ingredients: half of a dried lotus leaf, one small handful of osmanthus blossoms, green tea, rock sugar

Method: ❶ Cut the dried lotus leaf into tiny pieces. Put them into a tea cup with osmanthus blossoms, green tea, and rock sugar. Pour in boiling

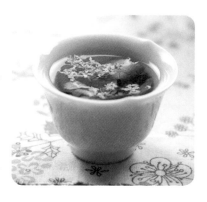

water. ❷ Cover and let it stand for five minutes before drinking.

Effects: Osmanthus tea can help the body expel toxins, balance the nervous system, and purify the body and mind.

Lotus Leaf and Watermelon Skin Tea

Ingredients: half of a dried lotus leaf, one piece of watermelon skin

Method: ❶ Wash the watermelon skin. Cut it into slices. ❷ Cut the dried lotus leaf into tiny pieces and put them into the pot with the watermelon skin. Decoct and get the juice.

Effects: In summer when the temperature is high, sports activities will accelerate the loss of water from the body, making heatstroke likely. At this time, drinking some lotus leaf watermelon skin tea can reduce heat and fats while generating saliva and quenching thirst.

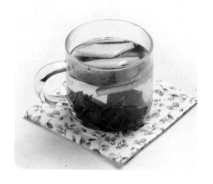

Lotus Leaf with Dried Tangerine Peel Oolong Tea

Ingredients: one dried lotus leaf, dried tangerine peel, oolong tea leaves

Method: ❶ Cut the dried lotus leaf into tiny pieces. Put them with the dried tangerine peel into a clay pot. Add water. ❷ Boil over a high heat. When it starts boiling, turn down the heat and continue brewing for 15 minutes. ❸ Put the oolong tea leaves in a cup. Pour in the soup and leave it to stand for three minutes.

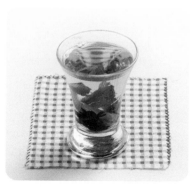

Effects: Both the tangerine peel and lotus leaf are effective at invigorating the spleen for eliminating dampness, and can expel dampness toxin from the body.

Barley Tea

Ingredient: one small handful of barley tea

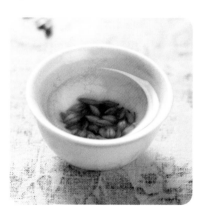

Method: ❶ Put the barley tea into a pot. Add water and bring to the boil. ❷ Turn off heat after 5 to 10 minutes. Drink after it has cooled down slightly.

Effects: Eating hot, spicy, and greasy food frequently will place a great burden on the stomach and spleen. Drinking barley tea can break down the grease and aid digestion, help the stomach and spleen to detoxify, and reduce physical discomfort.

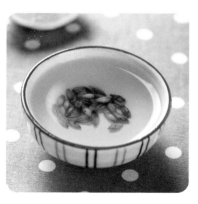

Barley and Lemon Tea

Ingredients: one small handful of barley tea, four cubes rock sugar, lemon juice

Method: ❶ Put the barley tea into a cup. Add boiling water. ❷ Keep it covered for three minutes. Add lemon juice. ❸ Add rock sugar. Stir gently.

Effects: Barley tea can invigorate the spleen, stimulate digestion, eliminate heat, and quench thirst. The high dietary fiber in barley tea means that it detoxifies and moistens the intestines. Barley tea is warm in nature. People whose stomach and spleen are cold and yet want to relieve constipation and lose weight can use barley tea instead of green tea, which has a cold nature.

Hawthorn and Lotus Leaf Tea

Ingredients: 15 slices hawthorn, one lotus leaf, two red dates

Method: ❶ Wash the lotus leaf. Tear into smaller pieces. Remove the pits from the red dates. Put them with the hawthorn and lotus leaf in a pot. Add water and bring to the boil. ❷ After five minutes, strain and then drink.

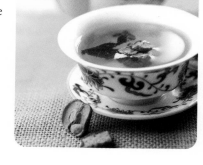

Effects: Hawthorn lowers blood lipids and blood pressure as well as dispersing *qi* and blood stasis. It is good food therapy for expelling heart and spleen toxins. Drinking hawthorn and lotus leaf tea regularly can also reduce fat and aid weight loss.

Hawthorn and Chrysanthemum Tea

Ingredients: three hawthorn slices, five chrysanthemum blossoms

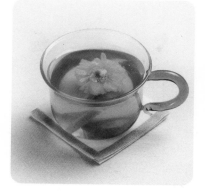

Method: ❶ Put the hawthorn and chrysanthemum in a cup together. Pour in boiling water. ❷ Keep it covered for ten minutes before drinking.

Effects: Hawthorn stimulates digestion and dissipates accumulated food. It should be noted that it tastes sour. To avoid excessive gastric acid secretion, it is not advisable to eat it on an empty stomach, especially for patients with gastric ulcers, as it may do more harm than good. To avoid adverse effects, it is advisable to eat hawthorn after dinner to strengthen the spleen and promote digestion.

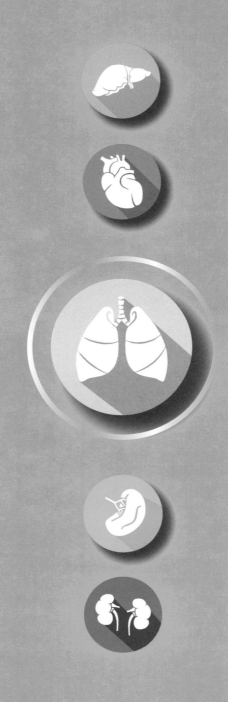

Chapter Five
Detoxifying the Lungs

Haze, secondhand smoke, and cooking fumes from the kitchen can cause serious damage to the lungs. In TCM theory, the heart governs the blood vessels and the lungs govern *qi*, but for the heart to govern the blood vessels, it requires *qi* to carry out its function. Similarly, in the process of digestion, absorption, metabolism, and nutrient distribution, the lungs also play a regulatory and controlling role.

The lungs are the heart's guardian. The heart needs the assistance of the lungs. The lungs nourish and regulate the various functions of the body through *qi*, disseminating the instructions, will, and spirit of the heart to wherever *qi* can reach, thus playing the role of governing, regulating, and exercising constraint to all life functions. Normally, the lungs will give accurate guidance and restraint to the heart, and will even rectify its mistakes, helping it to distribute blood to the rest of the body.

The overall *qi* in the body is controlled and regulated by the lungs. Along with the development of TCM, the concept of *qi* is constantly being extended and enriched. Sometimes, *qi* refers to energy, such as the cold, hot, warm and cooling nature of food or medicine. For example, after eating mutton, the body will feel hot, and if the amount consumed is too much, dry mouth and dry tongue syndrome will occur. The reason for this, according to TCM, is that mutton has a hot nature and can strengthen *yang qi*. The *qi* mentioned in TCM mainly comes from two aspects. First is the innate *qi* stored in the kidneys, which is from the parents' blood essence, and is genetic. The other is the nutrient essence generated by the spleen and stomach, as well as the environmental air inhaled through the lungs. The former provides conditions for the birth of life, while the latter provides nourishment and power for the growth of life. Therefore, the lungs dominate the whole body's *qi*, which includes the clean air that results from respiratory activities and directly affects the operation of the entire *qi* system. If the respiratory function of the lungs is normal, inhaled air is cleaned and dirty or impure air is exhaled, thus the acquired *qi* will be vigorous and abundant. However, if there is abnormality in the respiratory function of the lungs, clean air from inhalation (which is one of the different types of *qi*) will be reduced, and the expulsion of dirty air or impure *qi* will be disrupted, causing the acquired *qi* to be deficient and insufficient. Therefore, to nourish the acquired *qi*, we should not only strengthen the spleen and stomach, but also regulate the lung *qi*.

1. Are There Toxins in Your Lungs?

As we inhale and exhale, we carry out life's survival functions. The main function of the lungs is breathing. Many ailments are actually hints from the lungs.

Coughing and phlegm: When we inhale, the air enters the lungs first, and then is transported to various parts of the body for use. Some people have the habit of wearing masks when they go out, as their throats feel uncomfortable without them on. They feel like there is phlegm in their throats, but they cannot cough it out. This is a typical lung discomfort caused by air pollution. The lungs open at the nose[1]—the direct connection

---

[1] The lungs control respiration. The nose is the uppermost end of the respiratory tract, and is the pathway of respiration. The lungs connect with nature through the nose, and the channels of the lungs are also connected with the nose. The physiological and pathological conditions of the lungs can be reflected in the nose.

with the outside world. The skin and hair on the exterior of the body, ruled by the lungs, are susceptible to invasions of exogenous pathogens. The lungs are an important life channel, and cannot tolerate any obstruction when extracting the clean air (clean *qi*) inhaled through respiration and exhaling the dirty air (turbid *qi*). Coughing is not necessarily a bad thing. It is the body's natural protective response. When we cough, the phlegm turbidity in the lungs can be discharged to encourage *qi*. However, prolonged coughing can cause damage to the normal physiological structure of the lungs and injure them. In this situation, we need to carry out timely treatment to repair the damage. One convenient method is to stimulate the lung meridian.

Dull complexion and hair loss: According to TCM theory, the lungs govern the skin and hair[2]. The lungs can transport bodily fluids, and nutrient essence that has been absorbed, to all parts of the body, even to the body and hair, giving the skin a moist and radiant look, and making the hair soft and lustrous. The skin and hair are nourished by the lung *qi*. The skin and hair, including the sweat glands and other tissues, are the external surface of the body. Together, they are responsible for secreting sweat, moisturizing the skin, and resisting external pathogens. If the lung function is abnormal, the ability to secrete sweat, moisturize the skin, and resist external pathogens will be lowered, and naturally, the skin will be affected.

Low, weak, and hoarse voice: Many people have a low, weak voice, and are unable to hit the right note even when singing. They also lack impact when shouting. These people experience shortness of breath and fatigue, and seem tired and

---

[2] Skin and hair depend on the *qi* essence of the lungs for nourishment and warmth. The diffusion of *qi* and the opening and closing of the sweat glands in the skin and hair are also closely related to the dispersion function of the lungs.

depleted. According to TCM, the lungs control the voice. As such, people with sufficient lung *qi* have loud, powerful voices, while the voices of those with weak lung *qi* are low and weak. A blockage in the lungs will lead to hoarseness or voice loss. In addition, when you are sad, you should cry, as crying is a normal way of relieving emotional tension, which is beneficial to your health. However, if you cry too often, it will cause damage to your lungs. Meanwhile, to tonify the lungs and *qi*, consume often ginseng, American ginseng, *dang shen* (codonopsis pilosula), *tai zi shen* (pseudostellaria heterophylla), astragalus, white atractylodes rhizome, and Chinese yam.

Vulnerability to catching colds: There are people who fall sick easily when somebody around them has a cold. These people's lungs often suffer from external pathogenic invasion. They are prone to spontaneous sweating, night sweating, and frequently catch colds. The lungs open to the nose, and the nose is the channel for breathing in and out. Therefore, when the lung *qi* is in harmony and functioning well, the nose can distinguish fragrance and odor. On the other hand, if the lungs are not in good condition, nasal congestion, runny nose, and abnormalities in one's sense of smell will arise. People who prone to catching colds should exercise more to improve their immunity. Moreover, the lungs, being at the highest position in the chest, are like an umbrella, shielding the viscera from wind and rain. Any invasion of cold pathogens and over-consumption of cold drinks can cause harm to the lungs. The key to protecting the lungs and preventing catching colds is to regulate the body's internal cold and heat in a timely manner.

Constipation: The lungs control the ascending and descending flow of bodily fluids, distributing them to the viscera and meridians. When the large intestine is nourished by bodily fluids, defecation will be normal. However, if the large intestine does not receive nourishment, it will be dry, and this will affect defecation. The lungs and large intestine are closely related to each other, as the interior and exterior. If the lung's purifying

and descending function deteriorates[1], it will affect the large
intestine's releasing function, causing blockages and leading to
constipation. The best treatment is to ventilate the lungs and
regulate the flow of *qi*[2]. White radish is an adjuvant treatment
for constipation in elderly people. In cases of severe constipation,
eat half a raw white radish every day for one week, and you will
see a significant improvement.

2. Habits That Harm the Lungs

The lungs are the most delicate of the five *zang* organs. To
protect and nourish the lungs, they should be clean and moist,
and internal coldness and heat should be moderate—neither too
high nor too low. If the lungs are turbid rather than clear, *qi* will
have no place to reside, and bodily fluids will be lost, leading to
a *wei-qi* (defensive *qi*) deficiency and lack of nourishment for the
body surface, allowing external evil to take advantage and enter.

Lying down for too long, harming the lungs: TCM looks
at *qi* as the basis of the body. *Qi* belongs to *yang*, and is action-
loving, being dispersed all over the body. Therefore, under
normal circumstances, *qi* is constantly moving around the body.
If *qi* slows down or is obstructed, it becomes stagnated, which
itself is already a pathological state. Lying down is static, which
is the opposing state of movement. This is obviously contrary
to the physiological characteristics of the action-loving *qi*. Clean
air from the environment is diffused into the blood by the lungs,
and the turbid *qi* in the body is also discharged from the body
through the lungs. This life channel is dominated by movement.
The respiratory functions of people who lie down for a long time

---

[1] The loss of the purifying and descending ability of the lungs. The
lungs govern *qi*, control breathing, and regulate water channels,
ensuring that the purifying and descending functions are smooth.
[2] Releasing stagnant lung *qi* and making it work normally.

and move little will be weakened. This will lead to less intake of clear air and more accumulation of turbid *qi*, making them susceptible to ischemia and hypoxia.

It is very important to establish a proper bedtime routine according to the ancient Chinese zodiac, which recommends sleeping well at *zi shi* and *wu shi*. *Zi shi* (23:00 to 01:00 at night) is the time the body can nourish and replenish the *yin qi*, while *wu shi* (11:00 a.m. to 13:00 p.m.) is the time of the day when the *yang qi* in the natural world is most abundant. Just by taking a 20-minute rest break at this time, you can replenish the *yang qi* in your body.

Spending long hours in air-conditioned rooms: The lungs are delicate organs, and are regarded as clean and peaceful in TCM. They dominate the distribution of *qi*, and prefer moisture rather than dryness. Thus, the pathogenic factors in the natural environment that can harm the lungs are dryness and heat. In autumn, dry air can invade the human body through the skin, body surface, mouth, and nose, and can dissipate bodily fluid, resulting in symptoms like dry mouth and tongue, dry skin and hair, decreased output of urine, and constipation. However, in modern life, environmental dryness and heat are not limited to autumn, but also occur in other seasons. Air conditioning has infiltrated modern life, and have become very popular, even though they cause a decline in environmental humidity. Moreover, bacteria from air-conditioning ventilation pipes will escape into the air through the opening, and people who breathe it in will naturally be infected.

Eating spicy and pungent food: According to TCM, spicy food enters the lungs, and moves *qi* and dissipates dampness. As such, it is more suitable for people who live in geographical basins, mountains, and humid places. However, if people living in dry areas consume a lot of spicy and pungent food, their bodily fluids will be seriously depleted in their lungs. Additionally, heavy drinking and talking or shouting will lead to a rapid loss of fluid in the nose, mouth, and trachea, resulting in insufficient bodily fluids and loss of support for the lungs. In autumn, the weather is cool, humidity is low, and the air is dry. It is at this time that symptoms such as dry throat and dry cough commonly occur. This is a phenomenon caused by dryness. At this time, consumption of spicy and pungent food should be cut down, as heat from these foods will aggravate lung dryness. Examples of this type of food are onion, ginger, and pepper.

An unhealthy and unrestrained diet: Irregular meals, frequent social activities, excessive drinking and eating meat are completely opposite to the principle of nourishing the lungs, and are not conducive to the detoxification of the kidneys. When the descending and purifying function of the lungs deteriorates, it can lead to insufficient kidney *yin* and kidney fluid. Over time, it will lead to a deficiency of kidney *yin*, dry skin, dry eyes and blurry vision, and shaky teeth and white hair, like plants after a long drought. If the foundation is not firm, the bones will not be strong, and weakening of the lower back and knees will soon occur. Hypertension, hyperglycemia, and hyperlipidemia are also related to this. Therefore, treatment for these diseases should incorporate some acupoint massage to regulate the lung *qi*, to strengthen its descending and purifying function and enhance the metabolism of energy. Important advice for asthmatic patients: Eat less food with a high fat content, but eat more pears, lychees, and white fungus. A research study showed that when asthmatic patients were given drug inhalers after eating a high-fat meal, their lung function improved by only 1%, while those who ate a low-fat meal improved by 4.5%.

3. Massage Therapy to Detoxify the Lungs

The Taiyin Meridians of the Hand pass through the lungs. In the five *zang* organs, the lungs govern *qi* and dominate breathing. In fact, the process of breathing, ascending/dispersing, and descending/purifying, is actually ventilating the lung *qi*.

Press the Chize Acupoint

Among the five elements, the lungs belong to metal. Fire can conquer metal, so lung ailments are most afraid of fire. In modern-day language, fire is inflammation. Therefore, TCM often treats such ailments by clearing away lung heat and expelling heat pathogens. If acupoints are used for treatment, select the Chize acupoint on the lung meridian.

In clinical practice, for any syndrome featuring lung heat obstruction (such as fever, cough, hemoptysis, yellow phlegm, asthma, and sore throat), performing the press-knead-tap manipulation on this point can effectively clear the lungs and relieve heat, moisten the throat, and ease swallowing.

After your shower, roll up a towel and hold it with one hand. Press it near the Chize acupoint on the opposite arm, and massage the arm in a circle to stimulate the point and the other nearby acupoints. Using the press-knead manipulation with your thumb on the Chize acupoint every day can enhance the function of your respiratory system and reduce the incidence rate of ailments such as coughing and asthma.

Acupoint location: On both arms. In the depression of the radial side of the biceps brachii tendon on the transverse line of the elbow.

Massage method: Bend your thumb, and press the Chize point with the pulp. Do this on both the left and right arms for three minutes each time at each point.

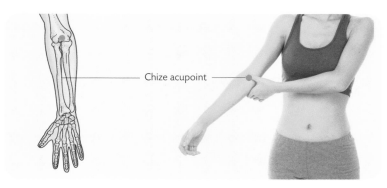

Chize acupoint

Press the Kongzui Acupoint

In case of an acute asthma attack, press-knead the Kongzui acupoint for several minutes to reduce and relieve the symptoms. When you catch a cold, you can use *gua sha* (scraping) therapy and scrape gently at and around the point for a few minutes. When the *sha*—a reddish skin rash comes up—the cold symptoms will be under control.

The Kongzui acupoint has another special function, namely to regulate the opening and closing of pores on the body's surface and the secretion of sweat. TCM perceives sweat as the bodily fluid released by the lung *qi*. Therefore, if the body is affected by external pathogens and a failure to disperse lung *qi*, it will lead to fever, aversion to cold, body pains, and no sweating. When this happens, you can massage the Kongzui acupoints to stimulate sweating and relieve the skin, as this will help to disperse lung *qi*.

Acupoint location: On the inner side of both forearms, 7 cun above the transverse crease of the wrist, and on the line joining the Chize and Taiyuan acupoints.

Massage method: Press the Kongzui acupoints with your thumb for three minutes each time.

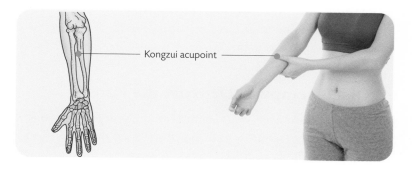

Kongzui acupoint

Press-Knead the Taiyuan Acupoint

The Taiyuan acupoint is the *shu* acupoint of the Taiyin Lung Meridian of Hand, and also the *yuan*-primary point of the lungs. According to the study of the meridians and collaterals,

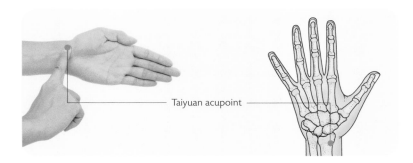

Taiyuan acupoint

shu acupoints are located near the wrist joints that irrigate and transport *qi* and blood. The *yuan*-primary point is the source of *qi* and blood, referring to the place where *yuan* (primordial) *qi* resides in the *zang-fu* and meridians. Therefore, stimulating Taiyuan acupoint can invigorate the *yuan qi* stored in the lung meridians and then transport it outward. It is also used to observe lesions on the lungs and the lung meridian in diagnosis.

Acupoint location: On both hands. At the wrist crease on the radial artery, between the styloid process of the radius and the navicular bone, and in the ulnar depression of the abductor pollicis longus tendon.

Massage method: To quickly relieve coughing and shortness of breath, press-knead the Taiyuan point with your thumb or index finger for three minutes until there is a feeling of tender swelling at the point.

4. Diet Therapy to Detoxify the Lungs

Breathing fresh air every day can improve the ventilatory system and enhance the respiratory exchange function of the lungs. Take walks and exercise in your local parks. You can care for your lungs by eating less spicy food, and include in your diet some food that clears away the lung-heat and moistens the lungs.

More Sour and Less Spicy Food
Spicy food disperses and promotes the circulation of *qi*. Most

spicy food can stimulate the appetite, invigorate the spleen and stomach. Spicy food enters the lungs and large intestine, and can encourage the dispersal and ascension of the lung *qi*. However, too much of it will have an adverse effect. TCM holds that an inappropriate diet is the main reason for autumn dryness, especially when the weather is dry. In autumn, people should use diet therapy to eliminate autumn dryness and nourish lung *yin*, for example, eating more *yin*-nourishing and moistening food such as pears, water chestnuts, honey, white fungus, apples, grapes, radish, lotus roots, lily bulbs, rock sugar, and duck.

Water chestnuts: Water chestnuts clear heat, generate fluid, cool the blood, and detoxify. They are rich in dietary fiber, and can encourage the metabolism of sugar, fats, and protein in the body.

Apples: The dietary fiber in apples can improve gastrointestinal peristalsis and detoxification.

Grapes: The fruit acid in grapes can encourage the gastrointestinal digestive function and maintain the balance of intestinal flora.

Lotus root: Lotus root is rich in dietary fiber and mucus protein. It can encourage intestinal peristalsis, helping toxins in the body to be excreted through feces. It can also inhibit the absorption of cholesterol, triglycerides, and other lipid substances.

Sour flavors restrain lung *qi* while pungent flavors disperse and purge the lung, so our diet should include more sour food and less spicy food. In autumn, the humidity in the air drops, giving this season the characteristics of dryness. Ailments related to dryness will occur in the lungs, skin, and large intestine. Therefore, it is advisable to eat sour fruit in autumn, such as hawthorn, lemons, grapefruit, and apples.

White Food

Most white foods (especially white fruits and vegetables) clear heat, encourage diuresis, clear the intestines, ease defecation, and eliminate phlegm.

Common white foods that have effective therapeutic properties are white radish and pear. According to TCM, white radish's sweet, pungent flavor and cooling nature enter the lungs and stomach meridian, and relieve blockages in the chest while relaxing the diaphragm. They strengthen the stomach and help digestion, eliminating phlegm and relieving coughing, moistening dryness and generating saliva, detoxifying and dispersing blood stasis, as well as clearing the bowels. Radish is especially suitable for people with emphysema and lung heat.

The consumption of pears to clear the lungs dates a long way back in Chinese history. According to TCM, pears are cold in nature and sweet in flavor. They enter the lung and stomach meridians. Pears generate saliva and relieve thirst, moistening the lungs and eliminating dryness, relieving coughing and phlegm, nourishing *yin* and reducing fire, and promoting swallowing. When eaten raw or juiced, they can clear away internal heat-fire, and treat ailments like sore throat, constipation, and dark yellow urine. Pear steamed with rock sugar can nourish *yin* and moisten your lungs, relieve coughing, clear phlegm, and protect your throat.

Delicious Healthy Recipes
Sautéed Sour and Sweet Beef with Scallion

Ingredients: 350 g beef tenderloin, 150 g onion, bell pepper, ginger, sugar, vinegar, cooking wine, soy sauce, scallion

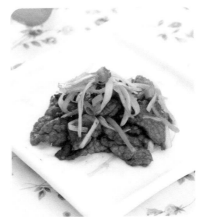

Method: ❶ Cut onions and ginger into strips. Remove the fascia from the tenderloin, wash and slice. Wash the bell pepper, and cut into strips. ❷ Marinate the beef with cooking wine, soy sauce, sugar, and ginger; mix everything

evenly. ❸ Heat the oil in a pan; add the beef with the onions and bell pepper. Add vinegar and sauté until cooked. Garnish with scallion.

Effects: Besides flavoring foods, the onion stimulates sweating, detoxifies, and promote the circulation of *yang qi*, as well as enhancing appetite.

Ginger and Red Date Porridge

Ingredients: 10 g ginger, 50 g round grain rice, five red dates

Method: ❶ Wash the rice. Chop up the ginger. ❷ Wash the red dates, and remove the pits. ❸ Put all the ingredients into a pot, add water, and boil until the porridge is cooked.

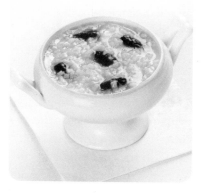

Effects: Ginger is warm in nature. It relieves abdominal distension, abdominal pain, diarrhea, and vomiting caused by excessive consumption of cold food. Add some ginger to the porridge to help expel pathogenic cold toxins and warm the stomach.

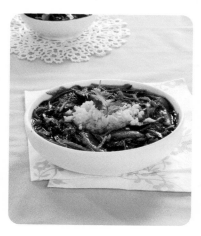

Eggplant with Garlic

Ingredients: one eggplant, half of a carrot, 15 g coriander, garlic, soy sauce, sesame oil, sugar, salt

Method: ❶ Wash the coriander, and cut into shorter sections. Wash the carrot, and cut into shreds. Mince the garlic. ❷ Soak the eggplant in salt water for five minutes. Remove from the water and cut into strips. Fry the eggplant strips in hot oil until soft. Dish out. ❸ Heat a little oil in the pan, and add the eggplant, carrot, soy sauce, sugar, and salt. Stir fry evenly until the flavors set in. Add sesame oil and garnish with coriander and minced garlic.

Effects: Garlic can relieve abdominal pain and whooping cough.

Coriander and Soybean Salad

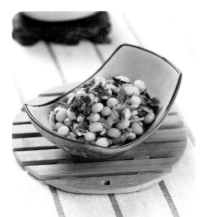

Ingredients: 20 g coriander, 50 g soybeans, Sichuan pepper, ginger, sesame oil, salt

Method: ❶ Wash the soybeans and soak them for more than six hours. Shred the ginger. ❷ Boil the soaked soybeans with the Sichuan pepper, ginger, and salt until cooked. Leave it aside to cool. ❸ Wash the coriander and cut. Mix in with the soybeans. Add sesame oil to taste.

Effects: Coriander has a spicy, pungent flavor. Spice stimulates the ascending function while pungency encourages the dispersion function. With these effects, coriander can help detoxify the lungs and spleen. Adding a little coriander to home cooking can enhance the flavor. Eating it often can encourage appetite, stimulate the stomach, and invigorate the spleen.

Lemon Rice

Ingredients: 200 g round grain rice, one lemon, salt

Method: ❶ Wash the lemon. Cut it in half. Slice one of the halves and mince the other one. ❷ Wash the rice. Add water and salt, and cook. ❸ After the rice is cooked, dish it up on a plate and sprinkle the minced lemon pieces on it. Decorate the side of the plate by laying the sliced lemon pieces around it.

Effects: When the weather is hot and humid, an inappropriate diet will lead to an accumulation of moisture in the body, which will generate phlegm. If phlegm accompanies a cough and a sore throat, eat lemon rice as your staple food to regulate and effectively expel dampness.

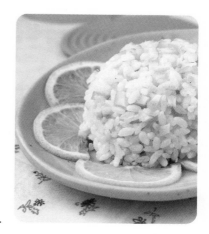

Apple and Corn Soup

Ingredients: two apples, one corn, salt

Method: ❶ Wash the apples and corn separately. Cut into small pieces. ❷ Put the apple and corn pieces into a pot, add water, and bring to the boil over a high heat. ❸ Turn the heat down and simmer for 30 minutes. Add salt to taste.

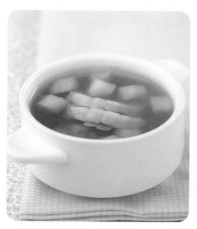

Effects: Apples taste sweet and slightly sour. They can help detoxify the lungs as they encourage saliva, relieve thirst, moisten the lungs and uplift moods, strengthening the spleen and stomach, nourishing the heart and *qi*, moistening the intestines, and stopping diarrhea. Apples can also improve skin elasticity and hydration, making it moister.

Pork and Radish Soup

Ingredients: 300 g pork, 200 g radish, scallion, ginger, salt

Method: ❶ Wash and cut pork and radish into smaller pieces. ❷ Heat the oil in a pan. Sauté the scallion and ginger. Add pork pieces and continue frying. Add salt to taste. ❸ Add a little water, and when it comes to the boil, turn the heat down and stew until the pork is soft.
❹ Add radish, and continue to stew until it is cooked and soft.

Effects: In winter, people often experience symptoms of lung toxicity such as dryness-heat, phlegm, and coughing. Pork and radish soup moistens the lungs, relieves coughing, and warms and nourishes the body.

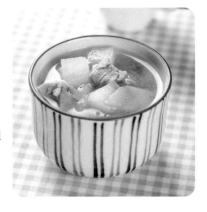

White Fungus Soup

Ingredients: 50 g white fungus, cherries, strawberries, walnuts, rock sugar, starch

Method: ❶ Wash the white fungus, and cut into tiny pieces. Wash the cherries and strawberries separately. Cut the strawberries in half. ❷ Cook the white fungus over a high heat, then turn down the heat and continue cooking for 30 minutes. Add rock sugar and starch and cook for a few more minutes. ❸ Add the cherries, strawberries, and walnuts. Turn off the heat once it starts to boil. Leave it to cool before eating.

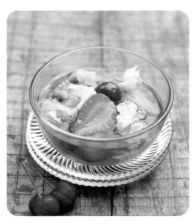

Effects: White fungus can strengthen bodily essence and tonify the kidneys. It can also nourish *yin* and moisten the lungs as well as supplementing *qi* and blood.

Onion Soup

Ingredients: 300 ml fresh milk, one onion, salt

Method: ❶ Remove the onion stem, wash, and cut into thin strips. **❷** Heat the oil in a pan. Sauté the onions, and add water. Lower the heat and simmer. **❸** When the onions are soft, add milk. When it starts boiling, add salt to taste.

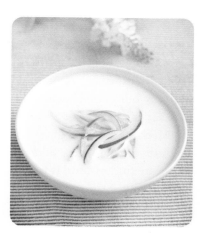

Effects: Milk can replenish deficiencies, invigorate the spleen and stomach, generate bodily fluids, and moisten the intestines. It can also encourage the expulsion of toxins in the intestines. Children and the elderly should drink more milk to strengthen their bodies.

Lotus Root with Rock Sugar

Ingredients: one segment of lotus root, 20 g wolfberry, pineapple, rock sugar

Method: ❶ Wash the

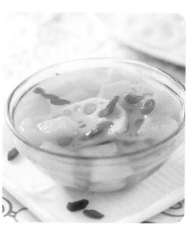

lotus root and pineapple separately. Peel and slice the lotus root. Cut the pineapple into pieces. Wash the wolfberries. **❷** Put the lotus root slices, pineapple pieces, and rock sugar into a pot. Add water and boil. **❸** When it is almost cooked, add the wolfberries. Boil until cooked.

Effects: Raw lotus root can clear heat, moisten the lungs, cool the blood, and remove blood stasis. It is effective at expelling lung toxins and blood stasis toxins. People with colds and coughs should try this dish.

White fungus, Lily and Soybean Milk

Ingredients: 60 g soybeans, 10 g each of white fungus and fresh lily bulbs, one banana, rock sugar

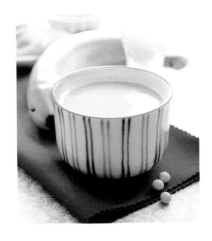

Method: ❶ Soak the soybeans for ten hours. Soak the white fungus until it is fluffy. Remove the old roots and other foreign substances. Tear into small florets. Break up the fleshy leaves of the lily bulbs. Wash and remove the roots. Peel the banana. Cut into smaller pieces. ❷ Put the soybeans, white fungus, lily bulbs, and banana into a soybean machine. Add water and start the machine. Strain. Add rock sugar and mix well. (If the soybean machine does not have a cooking function, precook the soybeans, white fungus and lily bulbs.)

Effects: Lily bulbs moisten dryness and clear heat. They can expel lung and heat toxins, and are often used to relieve symptoms such as lung dryness and coughing.

Chinese Yam with Chicken Congee

Ingredients: 100 g each of Chinese yam, round grain rice, and chicken breast, celery, cooking wine, salt

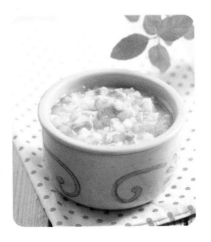

Method: ❶ Wash the Chinese yam, peel the skin off, and dice it. Wash the celery and dice it. ❷ Mince the chicken breast, add cooking wine, and mix evenly. ❸ Wash the round

grain rice, add water, and boil. When the congee is almost ready, add the Chinese yam, celery, and chicken mince. Cook for another ten minutes. Add salt to taste.

Effects: Chinese yam can strengthen the spleen, replenish *qi,* and relieve coughing and asthma. In autumn and winter when colds are frequent, consuming it can expel lung toxins.

Oatmeal Brown Rice Paste

Ingredients: 40 g oats, 30 g brown rice, 20 g black sesame, 15 g red dates, wolfberries, small pieces of rock sugar

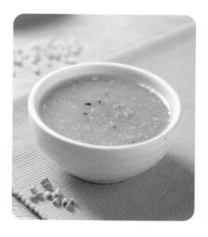

Method: ❶ Wash the brown rice and soak in water for ten hours. ❷ Wash the wolfberries, oats, and red dates separately. Remove the pits from the red dates. ❸ Put all the ingredients into a soybean machine except the rock sugar. Add water. ❹ Start the machine and make the mixture into a paste. Pour out the paste and add rock sugar to taste. (If the soybean machine does not have a cooking function, cook all the ingredients beforehand.)

Effects: Oats have high nutritional value, and have a positive effect on the complexion. They can increase skin vibrancy, reduce wrinkles, and remove pigmentation caused by toxin deposits.

Grapefruit Celery Juice

Ingredients: one stalk of celery, half a grapefruit, half a carrot

Method: ❶ Trim off the withered celery leaves. Wash and cut it into short sections. ❷ Wash the carrot and grapefruit separately. Remove the skin and cut into smaller pieces. ❸ Put the celery, carrot, and grapefruit into a juicer. Add water and start the juicer.

Effects: Studies have found that people who drink grapefruit juice every day rarely have respiratory ailments. This drink is especially effective at relieving toxic pulmonary ailments such as colds and sore throats.

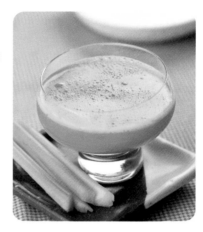

Mango and Orange Juice

Ingredients: one mango, one orange

Method: ❶ Wash the mango, peel, and remove the pit. ❷ Wash the orange, and remove the peel and seeds. ❸ Cut the mango and orange pulp into smaller pieces. Put in a juicer. Strain the juice when it is done.

Effects: According to TCM, oranges are sweet and sour in flavor, and can enter the lung meridian. They promote the secretion of saliva and body fluid, relieve thirst, and stimulate the stomach, moving *qi* downwards. For patients with bronchitis, oranges are effective at expelling lung toxins.

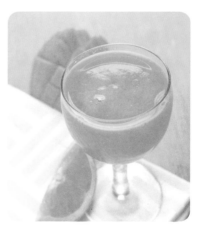

5. Tea Therapy to Detoxify the Lungs

Ailments like coughing, phlegm, and discomfort in the throat indicate that the lungs may not be in very good condition. People are now paying more attention to the health of their lungs, especially with air pollution becoming more severe. TCM holds that the lungs control the skin, so if the lungs are well, the skin is good. If you want your skin to be moist, eat more lung-nourishing food. Try the following tea recipes to moisten your lungs. You will find that your skin feels less dry and your throat does not ache.

Lily and Longan Tea

Ingredients: three edible lily blossoms, three longans, date kernels, honey

Method: ❶ Put the pulp of the longans with the lily blossoms and date kernels in a cup. ❷ Pour boiling water into the cup and soak the ingredients for ten minutes. Add honey, and mix well.

Effects: Lily blossom moistens the lungs, relieves coughing, and calms the heart and mind. When eaten often, it can also detoxify and improve the complexion.

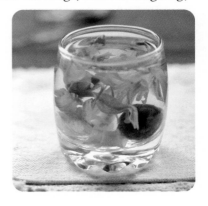

Almond and Chrysanthemum Tea

Ingredients: five bitter almonds, four dried chrysanthemum blossoms, honeysuckle, honey

Method: ❶ Put the bitter almonds, chrysanthemum, and honeysuckle in a cup. Pour in boiling water. ❷ Cover the cup. Leave it for five minutes. Add honey. Mix well.

Effects: Drinking almond chrysanthemum tea frequently can improve the body's immunity and resist wind pathogens.

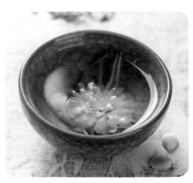

Almond Tea

Ingredients: eight sweet almonds, three bitter almonds

Method: ❶ Wash the sweet and bitter almonds separately. Pound them to pieces. ❷ Put them in a teapot. Add boiling water. ❸ Leave in the teapot for 20 minutes, then drink.

Effects: Eating almonds frequently can moisturize the lungs, and nourish and condition the skin, making it moist and give it radiance.

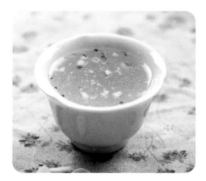

Lily and Peach Blossom Tea

Ingredients: three edible lily blossoms, two dried peach blossoms, one slice lemon

Method: ❶ Put the lily and peach blossoms into a cup. Pour in boiling water. ❷ Cover the cup. Leave it to stand for five minutes.

Effects: One of the possible causes of acne outbreaks on the face may be excessive fire in the

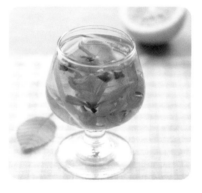

heart[1]. Peach blossoms can nourish the heart and calm the mind, and lily flowers can moisten the lungs and reduce inflammation. Both can help the body expel heart and lung toxins, and can make the skin smooth, even, and silky.

---

[1] A deficiency of heart *yin* and hyperactive interior generated by deficient fire. The main manifestations in clinical studies include insomnia, incoherent speech, and ulcers on the mouth and tongue.

Luo Han Guo (Dried Monk's Fruit) Tea

Ingredient: half a *luo han guo*

Method: ❶ Wash the *luo han guo*, remove the shell, and break into tiny pieces. Put the pieces into a cup. **❷** Pour boiling water into the cup and keep it covered for ten minutes.

Effects: Long-term smokers, people who use their voice excessively, and those who often stay up late should consume *luo han guo* to eliminate lung toxicity. Iced *luo han guo* tea is very refreshing for the mind, and stimulates the production of bodily fluids. It also prevents respiratory tract infections.

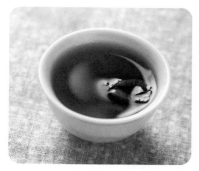

Luo Han Guo and Hawthorn Tea

Ingredients: one *luo han guo*, five slices hawthorn

Method: ❶ Wash the *luo han guo*, remove the shell, and put it in a pot with the hawthorn slices. **❷** Add an appropriate amount of water, and boil over a high heat. When it starts boiling, lower the heat and continue cooking for five minutes. **❸** Drink when it has cooled to a suitable temperature.

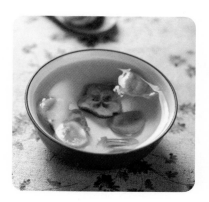

Effects: *Luo han guo* enters the lung meridian and the large intestine meridian. It moistens the lungs, relieves cough, generates saliva, and relieves thirst while moistening the intestines. For issues such as thirst, laryngitis, and tonsillitis, you can make *luo han guo* tea and soup.

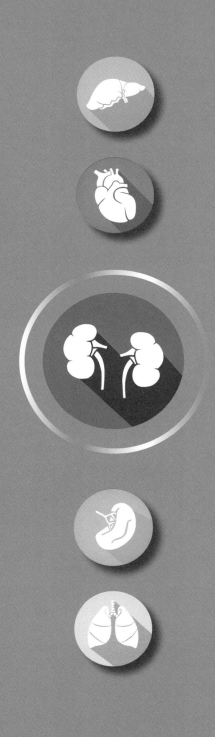

Chapter Six
Detoxifying the Kidneys

Of the five *zang* organs, the kidneys belong to the water element, and are the root of life. A tree, no matter how luxuriant it is, needs to hide its roots. Only if the roots are well hidden can they be taken out when needed. Similarly, the kidneys govern storage.

The kidneys store essential *qi*[1] and nourish the viscera. Their main function is to store and seal essential *qi* in the body. Essences functionally refer to all the essential substances in the body, such as *qi*, blood, bodily fluids, and nutrition from water and grain. They are collectively referred to as essential *qi*. In a narrow sense, it refers to the essence of human reproduction. As for its source, our innate essence comes from our parents, and our acquired essence comes from nutrient of food and drink transformed by the spleen and stomach. Therefore, in TCM, essence is the basic material that constitutes the human body and encourages human life activities. It is sealed in the kidneys for growth, development, and reproduction. Only when the kidneys are full of *qi* can a person be strong, agile, and energetic enough to continue life and reproduce.

The *qi* generated from kidney essence[2] directly determines the growth, development, and reproductive ability of human beings. When you are young, your kidneys are full of energy.

---

[1] The essence and *qi* of the body.

[2] The essence in the kidneys comes from the innate essence, and depends on the nourishment of the acquired essence, which is the material basis for the functional activities of the kidneys.

Men discharge semen, and women menstruate to reproduce. As we age, the essence in the kidneys will gradually decline, leading to gradual dwindling of sexual function and fertility of people until it totally disappears.

The kidneys are the base for sealing and storage, and thus store essence. The strength of their storage function directly affects the opening and closing of the urethra, vagina, and anus. Therefore, the treatment of urinary incontinence or retention, abnormal fecal excretion, male spermatorrhea and premature ejaculation, as well as women's leukorrhea often starts with the kidneys in TCM.

TCM regards the kidneys as the origin of congenital constitution, and the source of life. Our *yang qi* is mainly inborn, so it has a lot to do with innate nature. The functionality and decline of *yang qi* is closely related to the state of the kidney *qi*. Therefore, our growth, reproduction, physical strength, and life span are all related to the kidneys.

1. Are There Toxins in Your Kidneys?

The kidneys are inextricably linked to menstruation, sexual function, and childbirth. If they are not in good shape, these physical functions will be affected. When these effects are manifested on the body surface, we must pay attention and make an effort to manage them.

Dark circles and lethargy: According to TCM theory, the kidneys govern water transportation, and manage the transformation and movement of bodily fluids. When the kidneys accumulate toxins, their function will be damaged and their ability to discharge excess fluid will be reduced. Manifestations will be dark circles on the eyes and edema on the body, and symptoms will be especially serious on the face. When there is a dysfunction in the kidneys, fluid metabolism will be impacted, leading to a difficulty in discharging waste materials. As a result, people will begin to feel low, and experience symptoms like fatigue and lethargy. When the body gives you these hints, do not take them lightly. One or two days of lethargy and fatigue can be resolved through sleep, exercise, and listening to music. However, if you are in this state for a long time, you must seek medical attention. Hot compresses can improve dark circles under the eyes. If you get up in the morning and realize you have dark circles under your eyes, you can rub your hands together until they are hot, and quickly press your eyes with the palms of your hand. Repeat this action more than ten times, several times a day.

Decreased menstrual flow, with a short duration and dark color: The generation and ceasing of menstruation, its duration, and the amount and color are all manifestations of kidney function. If there are many toxins in the kidney, the amount of menses will be reduced. Women with such symptoms should seek medical advice without delay. Adjust your diet to include foods that can tonify the kidneys as well as *qi* and blood. By regulating your menstrual cycle, you are adjusting your physiological state. Keep your body warm if your flow is not smooth. Kidney deficiency and insufficient blood and essence will lead to light periods, allowing the cold and cold pathogens to invade the body. When the blood is cold and stagnant, menses will not flow smoothly. Therefore, take care of your kidneys by keeping warm.

Heavy hair loss: The growth and nourishment of hair depend on the essence in the kidneys, and the blood. There are many reasons for hair loss, including a deficiency or an excess, or a combination of both, but it is mostly due to a deficiency of liver and kidney *yin*. Young and middle-aged people with full blood and essence have hair that is long and shiny. Conversely, old people's blood and essence is weak, and experiences deficiency, so their hair turns white and falls out. However, for some people who suffer premature hair loss, their hair becomes dry and brittle, grays prematurely, and eventually falls out. Such symptoms are related to insufficient essential *qi* and deficiency of blood in the kidneys. To have healthy hair, it is necessary to nourish the kidneys and liver. To treat hair loss and gray hair, you need to nourish the liver and replenish blood. Add more food to your diet that can nourish the kidneys and liver. Treat these two *zang* organs together as they support each other, adjusted according to each patient's degree of deficiency and need, and you will achieve greater results.

Lumbago: Lower back pain is usually due to a kidney deficiency or insufficiency of kidney *qi*. If it is accompanied by dizziness and tinnitus, it is necessary to seek timely medical attention, as this is not merely physiological pain caused by exercise or labor.

2. Habits That Harm the Kidneys

Although it is common knowledge that long-term drinking harms the kidneys, few people can stop. If you want to maintain your health, you should also avoid the following bad habits.

A prolonged bad sitting posture: The position of the spinal cord in modern medicine is the main route of the Du Meridian in TCM. The Du Meridian closely connects the brain and the root of life—the kidneys. Any injury to the bone marrow and spinal cord may appear to be harming the bone marrow, neck, chest, and lower back only. However, in fact, it is the kidney *qi* that is ultimately injured. According to TCM theory, the bones and spine are transformed by kidney essence. Their growth, development, and restoration require the kidney essence to nourish and replenish. The bone ridge is the natural extension and expansion of kidney *qi*. Therefore, if bones are injured by external forces or disease, the injury will inevitably enter and harm the kidneys. Therefore, avoid sitting for a long time, and massage yourself frequently instead. When you have been sitting for 40 minutes to an hour, stand up and stretch, do some kicking motions with your legs, or hold your hands behind your back, interlock your fingers, and beat your lower back muscles.

When you are in bed at night, massage your lower back. Do this persistently over a period of time, as it is good for the kidneys.

Excessive use of the brain: TCM has attributed the majority of mental function, thinking, and consciousness to the heart, while modern science believes that these functions belong to the brain. In fact, these two lines of thinking do not contradict each other. TCM holds that the brain is a sea of marrow. Marrow is born in the kidneys. As the highest form of human activity, its material basis is essence and blood. The essence is stored in the kidney, and the blood is controlled by the heart and transformed by the essence. *Jing shen* (spirit) is *jing* (essence) followed by *shen* (mind). Therefore, the mental activities and intellectual part of the heart need coordination between the heart and kidneys[1] in order to function properly. After high-intensity mental work, the first way to recuperate is through sleep. Rest relieves fatigue of the brain and strengthens the digestive function of the spleen and stomach. Another way is through physical exercise, which is a form of physical labor. In fact, physical strength and mental strength have a mutually neutralizing effect.

Sexual activity after drinking: After drinking, the liver and kidneys are in a state of deficiency. If you have sexual activity at this time, your energy level, which may not be as strong as before drinking, may be weakened further. This is a taboo for health maintenance. Binge drinking is one of the main issues in the theoretical system of TCM. Clinically, impotence, premature ejaculation, and irregular menstruation are often related to sex after drinking. Modern medicine believes that long-term sexual

---

[1] There is a cohesive and balanced relationship between heart and kidneys. The heart in the upper *jiao* belongs to the fire element. The kidneys are in the lower *jiao* and belong to the water element. The heart fire descends on the kidney, warming the kidney fluid. The kidney fluid helps the heart, nourishes the heart *yin*, restricts the heart *yang*, and stops the heart *yang* becoming hyperactive.

intercourse when inebriated will weaken the regulatory function of the immune system.

Abuse of kidney tonifying drugs: According to TCM, kidney *qi* damage can be due to a congenital deficiency, lack of nourishment after birth, imbalance from prolonged illness, or overwork, resulting in kidney deficiency. To tonify the kidneys, it is very important to distinguish between *yin* and *yang*, otherwise the result may be more harmful than beneficial. The main characteristic of TCM is the emphasis on differentiating deficiencies and needs based on the congenital constitution of each individual. Kidney deficiency is either *yin* or *yang* deficiency. Each category has its own treatment principles. Therefore, even the most common kidney tonic may not be suitable for everyone.

Frequent holding of urine: Restraining urination is very common, especially for students, drivers, and tourists. However, there is a degree of harm in holding back urine. A less severe case is urinary tract infection, and more severe cases can lead to renal failure. Clinically, patients with urinary tract infections often miss out on the best cure due to untimely and incomplete early treatment, which seriously affects the renal function. People who often hold their urine should immediately change their habits. Those who suffer from urinary tract infections must also stop holding their urine, in addition seeking medication from their doctor.

3. Massage Therapy to Detoxify the Kidneys

Both men and women should take good care of their kidneys. The following recommended massages are simple, safe, and reliable for young, middle-aged, and elderly people to carry out in their spare time.

Press-Knead the Zhaohai Acupoint
The Zhaohai acupoint belongs to the Shaoyin Kidney Meridian of Foot. It nourishes *yin* and reduces fire, tonifies the kidney *qi*,

and regulates the *san jiao* (triple warmer)[1]. It is also involved
in the balance of *yin* and *yang*. The Zhaohai acupoint can also
calm the mind and enhance sleep. The kidneys and bladder in
the five *zang* organs and six *fu* organs, as well as the Shaoyin
kidney meridian and the Taiyang bladder meridian, have similar
exterior and interior relation[2] and *yin-yang* relation. Therefore,
the TCM way of purging excesses[3] in the kidney meridian
is usually to go through the bladder meridian. Therefore, in
clinical practice, the Zhaohai acupoint or Shenmai acupoint on
the bladder meridian can be used to treat throat dryness, pain
and discomfort, hoarseness, insomnia, edema, urinary retention,
urinary tract infection, irregular menstruation, vaginal discharge,
and priapism.

   Acupoint location: On both feet. One cun below the tip of

---

[1] The combined name of the upper, middle, and lower *jiao*. It is a
   division of the body cavity, and a functional concept as one of the six
   fu organs. In terms of location, the upper *jiao* generally refers to the
   part above the chest diaphragm, including the heart and lungs. The
   middle *jiao* refers to the parts below the diaphragm and above the
   umbilicus, including the spleen and stomach. The lower *jiao* refers to
   the part below the umbilicus, including the kidneys, bladder, small
   intestine, and large intestine.

[2] The *yin* and *yang* meridians among the twelve meridians are
   interrelated and cooperate with each other, forming a relationship
   of external and internal integration. namely: the hand Taiyin and
   hand Yangming, the hand Jueyin and hand Shaoyang, the hand
   Shaoyin and hand Taiyang, the foot Taiyin and foot Yangming, the
   foot Jueyin and foot Shaoyang, the foot Shaoyin and foot Taiyang—
   six pairs of hands and feet altogether. The *yin* meridian belongs to
   the interior, and the *yang* meridian belongs to the exterior. The two
   meridians, which are external and internal to each other, follow the
   relative positions of the inner and outer sides of the limbs, and meet
   at the ends of the limbs.

[3] Dispelling pathogens. There is also tonifying deficiency, that is,
   nourishing the healthy *qi* of the body.

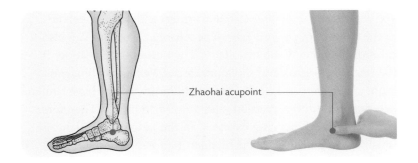

Zhaohai acupoint

the medial malleolus, in the marginal depression.

Massage method: Press and knead the Zhaohai acupoints gently with the pulp of your finger for three minutes each time, to tonify the kidneys, nourish the liver, and strengthen the spleen.

Scrape the Taixi Acupoint

In the study of meridians, the Taixi acupoint is a *shu* acupoint on the Shaoyin Kidney Meridian of Foot, and also the *yuan*-source point[1] for the kidneys. *Shu* acupoint is the place where this particular meridian and meridian-*qi* converge, and its role is to transport out the essence of Shaoyin and nourish *yin* and the kidneys. The *yuan*-source point is the place where the primordial *qi* (*yuan qi*)[2] in the kidneys resides. According to TCM, *qi* (especially the primordial *qi* in the kidneys) is the power source that propels the life activities of the human body. As such,

---

[1] The twelve meridians have important acupoints near the wrist and ankle joints. Each of the twelve meridians has one *yuan*-source point, which is the place where the vital energy of the *zang-fu* organs passes through and gathers.

[2] Primordial *qi* is innate. It is hidden in the kidneys, and depends on the acquired essence for nourishment. It is the basic material and motive force for maintaining human life activities. Its main functions are to support the growth and development of the body, and to warm and stimulate the physiological functions of the viscera, meridians, and other tissues and organs.

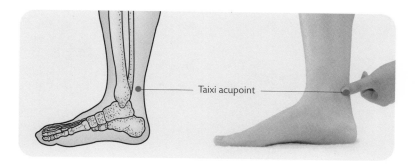

Taixi acupoint

this point plays a very important role in the kidney meridian. Moreover, the Taixi acupoint is a combination of two acupoints, with the *qi* of the kidney meridian being the most abundant. It nourishes kidney *yin*, tonifies the kidney *qi*, strengthens the kidney *yang*, and regulates the uterus. In other words, the Taixi acupoint can be the point of treatment for all types of kidney deficiency.

Acupoint location: On both feet. At the ankle area, in the depression between inner ankle tip and the Achilles tendon.

Massage method: Scrape the Taixi acupoints from top to bottom with the pulp of your finger for three minutes every morning and evening. This will regulate and alleviate nephritis, cystitis, enuresis, and spermatorrhea.

Massage the Yongquan Acupoint

Water is the source of life and the fundamental guarantee for human survival and health. No one can live without it. The Yongquan acupoint is the "well point" of the Shaoyin Kidney Meridian of Foot. The acupoints that are called "well" are all located at the ends of the limbs, like springs that have just sprung up from the ground. As the root of the body's *yin* and *yang*, essence and blood, the kidney meridians start from the sole of the foot, where the water of life gushes, metaphorically speaking. Using the pushing and kneading manipulation on the Yongquan acupoint can treat coma, shock, and asphyxia. It can relieve headaches, dizziness, mental malaise, and hypertension.

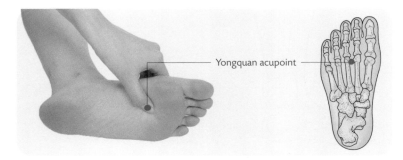

Yongquan acupoint

It can also alleviate palpitations, insomnia, and sore throats. Dry, rough, and aging skin, frostbite, and chapped feet can also benefit when this point is massaged. The treatment point for impotence, spermatorrhea, and infertility is also on the Yongquan acupoint.

Acupoint location: On the sole of both feet, at the most concave part of the center when you bend your toes.

Massage method: Rub and tap the Yongquan acupoints with your palm, or press-knead them with your thumb until your feet feel warm.

4. Diet Therapy to Detoxify the Kidneys

TCM stresses the homology of medicine and food. The healthcare and wellness doctrine that has lasted for thousands of years has all the information we need to study and learn how to improve the kidneys with food.

Salty Food

The kidneys have the function of regulating water metabolism. Taking in an appropriate amount of salty food can strengthen the kidney *qi*. Salty food can regulate the osmotic pressure balance of human cells and blood and the metabolism of water and salt, and can enhance physical strength and appetite. Therefore, drinking some salt water after vomiting, diarrhea, and excessive sweating can prevent a lack of trace elements in the body.

However, salty food should be eaten at a moderation, and not too much. The World Health Organization recommends that the intake of salt should be less than 6 grams per person per day. A long-term high-salt diet will lead to cardiovascular and cerebrovascular diseases, diabetes, and hypertension. About 80% of patients with renal diseases also have hypertension, and 80% of patients with renal diseases and hypertension suffer from volume-dependent hypertension, that is, the sodium ion concentration in their body is too high. Therefore, a low-salt diet is necessary for all patients with kidney diseases.

Too much salty food will lead to damage to the kidney *qi* and bones, muscle atrophy and weakness, chest tightness, and palpitations. Once a person's kidney *yang* is damaged, there will be a decline of the vital gate fire[1], followed by a suppression of their heart fire. Chaos and disorder will take place in the circulation of *qi*, blood, and bodily fluids, resulting in diseases. Cured food is high in sodium. Long-term consumption of such food will lead to excessive salt intake, which will affect the water/salt balance in the body, leading to blood pressure fluctuation, damage to kidney function, and an increased burden on the kidneys.

Black Food

Among the five *zang* organs, the heart dominates the spirit, and is nourished by the blood. At the same time, the kidneys also store essence and generate marrow, then transmit upward to the brain, thus becoming a repository for marrow. Therefore, as the "spirit" of the highest sort of human life activities, its most

---

[1] When kidney *yang* declines, it loses its ability to generate warmth, and lacks power to transform nutrients into *qi*, resulting in *yin*-cold excess, leading to a marked decline of sexual and reproductive functions.

important material basis is essence and blood, and essence can transform blood. Therefore, in TCM, it is believed that anything that can nourish the kidneys and generate essence nourishes the brain as well. The most famous kidney tonic is black sesame seeds. Black sesame is a good food for students and people who use their brains a lot. Grind black sesame seeds into powder, and mix with some glutinous rice flour and sugar to make homemade black sesame paste, which is a tonic for the brain as well as a simple breakfast food.

The color black governs water and enters the kidneys. Therefore, eating black food frequently can tonify the kidneys. Black sesame, edible fungus, and laver have high nutritional and medical value. They can significantly reduce the incidence of arteriosclerosis, coronary heart disease, and stroke, and have positive effects on influenza, chronic hepatitis, kidney disease, anemia, and hair loss. Black beans tonify the kidneys, strengthen the body, invigorate the spleen and promote diuresis, regulate the middle warmer and lower *qi*, encourage blood circulation and reduce swelling, moisturize dark hair, and enhance anti-aging. It is especially suitable for people with kidney deficiency or those with both spleen and kidney deficiency. Fermented black beans and tofu have a greater effect on tonifying the kidneys.

Delicious Healthy Recipes
Asparagus and Clam Rice

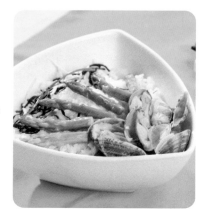

Ingredients: six asparagus stalks, 150 g clams, seaweed, round grain rice, ginger, bell peppers, sugar, vinegar, sesame oil, salt

Method: ❶ Wash the asparagus and cut it into shorter lengths. Cut the seaweed, ginger, and bell pepper into thin strips. Soak the clams in water; after they have purged out all the grit, cook them in water. Wash the round grain rice; transfer it to a rice cooker and add the appropriate amount of water. ❷ Mix the seaweed, ginger, and pepper strips with sugar, vinegar, and salt. Add them to the rice cooker. Place the asparagus on top and cook all of them together. When the rice is done, dish out. Add the clams and some sesame oil. Mix evenly.

Effects: Clams taste salty, which can generate bodily fluid, moisten the five *zang* organs, stop thirst, stimulate the stomach to enhance appetite, treat edema, and remove phlegm.

Oyster and Tofu Soup

Ingredients: 200 g each of oysters and tofu, scallions, garlic, cornstarch, shrimp stock, salt

Method: ❶ Wash the oyster meat and cut it into small pieces. Wash the tofu and cut it into cubes. Cut the scallions into thin strips and slice the garlic. ❷ Heat the oil in a pan, and sauté the garlic. Pour in the shrimp stock, add

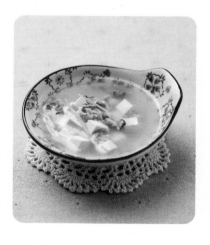

water, and bring to the boil. ❸ Add tofu and salt, and bring to the boil. Add the oyster meat, scallions, and starch (cornstarch mixed with water).

Effects: Oyster meat is a good tonic food for the kidneys. It has a positive effect on alleviating kidney toxin symptoms such as insomnia, dizziness, and headache caused by *yin* deficiency.

Millet and Sea Cucumber Porridge

Ingredients: 20 g dried sea cucumber, 80 g millet, wolfberries, salt

Method: ❶ Soak the dried sea cucumber until it expands. Remove the internal organs. Wash and cut it into shorter sections. **❷** Wash the millet, and soak for four hours. Add water and sea cucumber to cook. **❸** When the porridge is almost done, add wolfberries and cook for a few more minutes over a low heat. Add salt to taste.

Effects: Sea cucumber contains trace elements such as vanadium. It is a nourishing food for all ages as it participates in the transportation of iron in the blood and removes toxins from the blood.

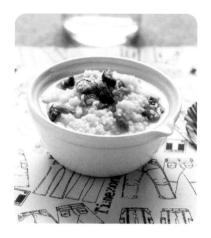

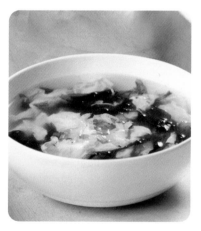

Small Dried Shrimp and Seaweed Soup

Ingredients: 10 g seaweed, one egg, small dried shrimps, scallions, ginger, sesame oil salt

Method: ❶ Wash the small dried shrimps. Break the seaweed into smaller pieces. Whisk the egg. Cut scallions and ginger into mince. **❷** Heat the oil in the pan, add the minced ginger, and small dried shrimps. Add water and bring to the boil. Pour in the egg mixture, add seaweed, salt, scallions and sesame oil.

Effects: Seaweed is rich in dietary fiber and minerals, which can help to discharge waste and toxins in the body. In this soup, seaweed and dried shrimps are supplements for iodine and calcium, and are ideal for students and people who use their brains a lot.

Kelp and Pine Nut Soup

Ingredients: 50 g pine nuts, 100 g kelp, chicken stock, salt

Method: ❶ Wash the pine nuts. Leave aside for later use. ❷ Wash the kelp. Soak in water for two hours. Cut into thin shreds. ❸ Pour in the chicken stock, pine nuts, and kelp shreds into a pot. Simmer over a low heat. Add salt to taste.

Effects: Kelp is very rich in iodine, which can strengthen the brain and improve intelligence. Kelp also contains a large amount of mannitol to reduce swelling and diuresis, and this helps to eliminate kidney toxins.

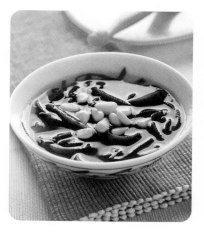

Indian Mustard and Dried Scallop Soup

Ingredients: 250 g Indian mustard, five dried scallops, chicken broth, sesame oil, salt

Method: ❶ Wash the Indian mustard, and cut into smaller sections. ❷ Soak the dried scallops in warm water for more than 12 hours. ❸ Wash the scallops, add water, and cook until soft. Shred the scallops. ❹ In a pot, add the chicken broth, Indian mustard, and scallop shreds, and cook. When the ingredients are cooked, add

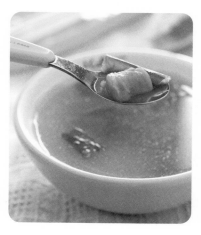

sesame oil and salt to taste.

Effects: Dried scallops can nourish *yin*, tonify the kidneys, and harmonize the stomach and the middle *jiao*[1]. It has a good detoxification effect on symptoms of kidney toxicity such as dizziness, weak spleen, and stomach.

Cucumber and Fungus Soup

Ingredients: 150 g cucumber, black fungus, salt

Method: ❶ Wash the cucumber and cut it into cubes. ❷ Soak the black fungus in cold water for six hours. Wash and remove the stems. ❸ Heat the oil in a pan, add the black fungus and stir fry, add water and bring to the boil. ❹ Put in the cucumber cubes. Add salt to taste.

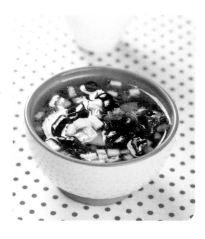

Effects: Black fungus is rich in iron. It is considered by nutritionists as a natural iron supplement, and purifies the blood. However, fungus has a cold nature, and it is not suitable for people with a weak spleen and stomach and bleeding diseases, nor is it good for those who have frequent diarrhea.

Fresh Lemon and Water Chestnut Drink

Ingredients: one fresh lemon, ten water chestnuts

Method: ❶ Wash the lemon, and slice it. ❷ Wash the water chestnuts. Peel and slice them. ❸ Add water to a pot, then add the lemon and water chestnut slices. Cook for 5 to 10 minutes.

Effects: Water chestnuts supplement *qi* and calm the middle

---

[1] Regulating the imbalance of stomach *qi* and the obstruction of middle *jiao*.

jiao, stimulating the appetite and digestion. They are also good for disease prevention, and are an antitoxic food. When eaten raw, they can spread bacteria and parasitic infection. Therefore, it is advisable to peel the water chestnuts and cook them for a little while in boiling water before eating.

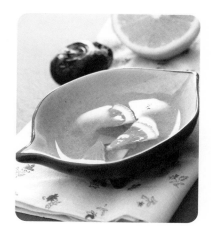

Black Sesame and Chestnut Paste

Ingredients: 40 g black sesame, 120 g cooked chestnuts

Method: ❶ Remove the shells of the cooked chestnuts. Peel the skin and cut into smaller pieces. **❷** Put the black sesame in a pot. Fry over a low heat until fragrant. **❸** Pour all the ingredients into a soybean machine. Add some water and beat it until a paste is formed. Garnish with some black sesame seeds.

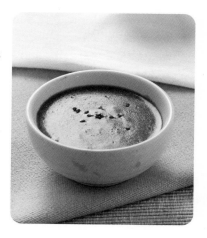

Effects: Eating black sesame is very good for detoxification and beauty.

Black Rice Paste

Ingredients: 50 g black rice, 30 g red beans, 25 g raw chestnuts, sugar, cooked sesame seeds

Method: ❶ Soak the red beans for ten hours. Remove the shells and skins of the chestnuts. Wash the chestnuts and black rice. Soak the rice for two hours. ❷ Put the red beans, chestnuts, and black rice into a soybean machine. ❸ After it has been made into paste, dish it out and add sugar to taste. Sprinkle some black sesame seeds. (In the absence of a soybean machine that has a cooking function, precook the black rice and red beans, and steam the chestnuts until cooked.)

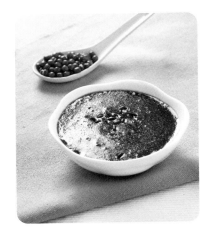

Effects: Black rice is rich in dietary fiber, which encourages gastrointestinal peristalsis and helps expel toxins.

Walnuts in Purple Rice Congee

Ingredients: 50 g purple rice, 50 g walnuts, 10 g wolfberries

Method: ❶ Wash the purple rice and soak for 30 minutes. Break the walnuts into smaller pieces. Remove impurities from wolfberries. Wash.

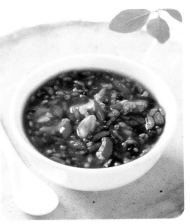

❷ Put the purple rice in the pot. Add water and bring to the boil. Cook over a high heat and when it boils, turn the heat down and continue cooking for 30 minutes. ❸ Add the walnuts and wolfberries. Continue cooking for another 15 minutes.

Effects: Both purple rice and walnuts have the effect of tonifying the kidneys. Purple rice is rich in dietary fiber, which can reduce the content of cholesterol in blood and help prevent heart diseases.

Mulberry Porridge
Ingredients: 50 g mulberry, 100 g glutinous rice, rock sugar

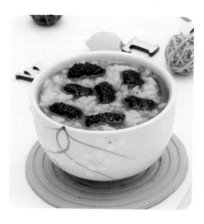

Method: ❶ Wash the mulberries. Wash the glutinous rice and soak for two hours. ❷ Put a pot on the stove. Add glutinous rice and water. Cook over a high heat. When it starts to boil, turn to low heat and continue cooking. ❸ When the porridge is soft and cooked, add the mulberries and cook for a few minutes. ❹ Add rock sugar. Mix well.

Effects: Mulberry can tonify the liver, nourish the kidneys, benefit the blood, and brighten the eyes. It has a curative effect on decreased visual acuity, tinnitus, physical weakness, and neurasthenia caused by a deficiency of liver and kidney *yin*.

5. Tea Therapy to Detoxify the Kidneys

When you begin to feel symptoms such as a worsening of the dark circles under your eyes, frequent backache, weakness when walking, or abnormal urination, it is your body telling you that your kidneys need to detox. When your kidneys are in good health, you will exude youth, vitality, and energy.

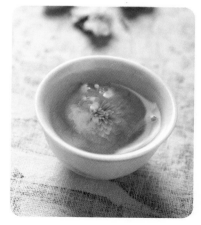

Wolfberry and Chrysanthemum Tea
Ingredients: five chrysanthemum blossoms,

six wolfberries

Method: ❶ Put the chrysanthemums and wolfberries into a cup. Pour boiling water. ❷ Let it stand for five minutes then drink.

Effects: Drink wolfberry chrysanthemum tea frequently to help the kidneys detoxify. It can also prevent and alleviate presbyopia and hearing loss due to old age.

Wolfberry and White Fungus Tea

Ingredients: one lobe of soaked white fungus, five chrysanthemum blossoms, wolfberries, rock sugar

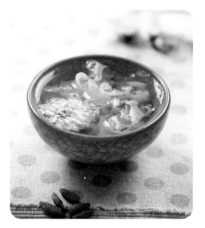

Method: ❶ Put the wolfberries, white fungus, and chrysanthemum in a pan. Add water. Cook over a low heat for 20 minutes. ❷ Turn off heat and add the rock sugar. When the rock sugar has melted, it is ready to drink.

Effects: Wolfberry is rich in β-carotene and can clear free radicals in the body as well as delaying the aging process.

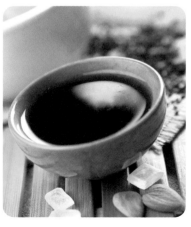

Black Sesame and Almond Tea

Ingredients: one small handful of black sesame seeds, five sweet almonds, green tea, rock sugar

Method: ❶ Mash the black sesame seeds and sweet almonds separately. ❷ Put all the ingredients in a cup. Add boiling water. ❸ Soak for five minutes. Stir to mix well, then drink.

Effects: Regular consumption of black sesame can replenish the kidneys and essence. As a result, it can expel kidney toxin and delay the aging process.

Black Sesame and Mulberry Leaf Tea

Ingredients: one small handful of black sesame seeds, five mulberry leaves

Method: ❶ Put the black sesame seeds and mulberry leaves in a cup. Pour boiling water into the cup. ❷ Leave it to stand for three minutes, then drink.

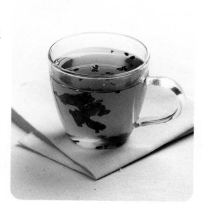

Effects: Excessive hair loss affects the appearance, and also signifies that the kidneys are overwhelmed. When too many toxins accumulate in the kidneys, it creates very unfavorable conditions for the kidney essence to generate blood. As a result, it loses its ability to nourish the hair. Therefore, it is advisable to eat food that nourishes the kidneys and benefits the essence. Black sesame seeds are one such food. They encourage the detoxification of the kidneys, restoring life and health to the hair.

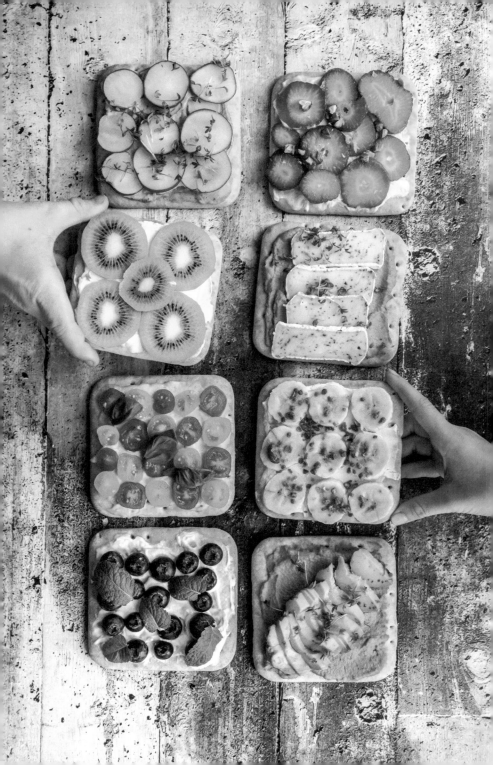

Chapter Seven
Detox Recipes for Everyone

Detoxification cannot be generalized. It is different from person to person. Whether for beauty or health care, as long as we persist in detoxification according to our individual needs, we will be energized and full of spirit, with healthy, youthful bodies.

1. Slimming Recipes for Women

After the age of 30, women begin to show signs of aging: eye bags, crow's feet, obvious skin pigmentation, getting out of shape, and more severe mood swings. When this happens, it is time to detoxify and regain your youth.

Detoxification through exercise: The main reason for detoxification through exercise is to increase oxygen in the blood, improve the metabolic rate, and speed up the discharge of carbon dioxide and other waste produced from carbohydrate and fat metabolism. Exercise can also encourage perspiration, which is quite helpful in strengthening the skin's detoxification function.

Detoxification through fasting: Include more cereals and vegetables in your diet; choose fresh fruits instead of fruit juice, and set aside one weekend every month for light fasting and detoxification at home. You can choose your preferred method, that is, eating only apples or bananas, or a stricter approach— fasting with water (Note: only people who have practiced light fasting long enough for their body to adapt to having no food should try water fasting), and then temporarily stop the use of skin care products to give your skin a chance to rest, so that your body can detoxify from the inside out.

Detoxification through sleep: This method sounds relaxing and comfortable. It is actually about the time you spend sleeping. The two most important detoxification organs in the body are the liver and the gallbladder, and they can only do their job when the body enters deep sleep.

Detoxification through food: Many foodstuffs have a detoxification effect as well as tasting good. For example, honey has a significant effect on moistening the lungs and relieving coughing, moistening the intestines and easing defecation, and detoxifying and enhancing the complexion. Cucumber can support metabolism and excrete toxins. Bitter gourd can expel heat, detoxify, enhance the vitality of the cortex, and make the skin silky and fine. Mung beans can clear internal heat, detoxify, relieve summer heat, and encourage diuresis, as well as significantly reducing fat. It also protects the liver and kidneys. The following are some recipes that can help women lose weight and enhance their looks.

White Fungus with Mung Bean Sprout Salad

Ingredients: mung bean sprouts, white fungus, green pepper, sesame oil, salt

Method: ❶ Wash the mung bean sprouts. Soak the white fungus until it expands. Wash and break into smaller pieces. Wash the green pepper. Cut it into thin shreds. ❷ Add water to a pot and bring to the

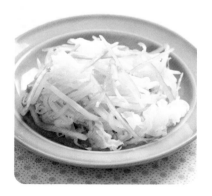

boil. Blanch the sprouts. ❸ Blanch the white fungus in boiling water until it is cooked. Put it in cold water. Drain dry. ❹ Lay the mung bean sprouts on a plate with the white fungus and green pepper shreds. Add sesame oil and salt. Mix evenly.

Effects: Regular consumption of white fungus can moisten the lungs, calm the dryness in the body, and help the lungs to detoxify.

Loofah Omelet

Ingredients: two eggs, one loofah, ginger, salt

Method: ❶ Wash the loofah. Peel and cut it obliquely. Blanch in boiling water. Mince the ginger. ❷ Add salt to the egg and beat. Fry it. Dish out. Heat the oil in a pan. Add ginger mince and sauté until fragrant. Put in the loofah pieces. Add salt to taste and stir fry. ❸ Turn up the heat to high and stir fry for a few more minutes. Add the fried egg. Stir fry a few more times.

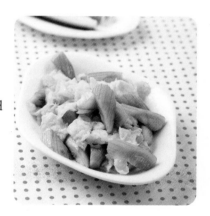

Effects: Eat loofah often, as it can make the skin smooth and delicate, reduce inflammation, expel toxins, and reduce melanin pigmentation.

Triple Vegetarian Joy

Ingredients: 200 g celtuce, 100 g carrot, 100 g radish, scallions, ginger, sesame oil, salt

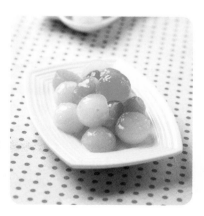

Method: ❶ Cut the scallions into short sections. Wash and peel the celtuce, carrot, and radish. Use a baller to shape them into balls. Blanch the balls thoroughly. ❷ Heat a little oil in a pan, put in scallions and ginger, sauté until golden, and dish out. Put water into a pot, put in the

celtuce, carrot, and radish balls until the water boils thoroughly. Turn the heat down and simmer for another few minutes. Add salt. Pour a little sesame oil over it.

    Effects: Eating more celtuce is recommended for people who suffer from frequent palpitations and insomnia, as it can reduce the load on the heart, relieve tension, and help sleep.

Black Sesame and Cabbage

Ingredients: 200 g cabbage, 30 g black sesame seeds, salt

    Method: ❶ Wash the cabbage, and cut into wide strips. Dry-fry black sesame seeds until fragrant and dish out. ❷ Heat the oil in a pan. Add cabbage strips. Stir fry several times. Add salt to taste. ❸ Stir fry until the cabbage is cooked and starting to turn soft. Dish out. Sprinkle black sesame seeds on it. Mix evenly.

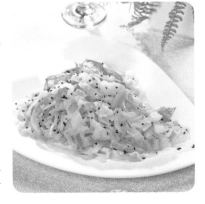

    Effects: Cabbage reduces internal heat and swelling, and has a detoxification effect. Regular consumption can expel toxins accumulated in the body and enhance immunity.

Pineapple and Bitter Gourd Juice

Ingredients: ¼ pineapple, ½ bitter gourd, ½ kiwi fruit, honey, salt

    Method: ❶ Wash the pineapple and kiwi fruit separately. Peel and cut into pieces. Wash the bitter gourd, remove the seeds, and cut into

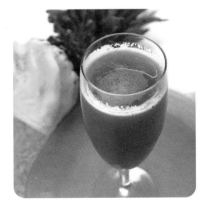

small pieces. ❷ Put the pineapple pieces into salt water, and soak for ten minutes. ❸ Put all the ingredients into the juicer and when it is done, add honey to taste.

Effects: Bitter gourd's rich nutrients include protein, vitamins, and minerals. Its unique components can regulate blood lipids and cholesterol, which is very beneficial to weight control.

Winter Melon and Honey Juice

Ingredients: 200 g winter melon, 20 ml honey

Method: ❶ Wash the winter melon. Remove its skin and cut into small pieces. ❷ Boil the winter melon in a pot of water for three minutes. Dish out and drain. Put the winter melon in a juicer, and add some water and juice. ❸ Add honey to taste. Stir to mix evenly.

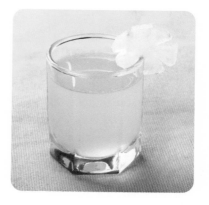

Effects: The reason why winter melon supports slimming through detoxification is that it can encourage diuresis and reduce edema. The tartronic acid in winter melon can inhibit the conversion of saccharides into fats and reduce the accumulation of fat. Moreover, winter melon is low in calories, and helps weight loss.

Tomato and Pomelo Juice

Ingredients: one tomato, four segments of pomelo

Method: ❶ Wash the tomatoes. Remove the pedicel and cut the tomato into small pieces. ❷ Remove the skin

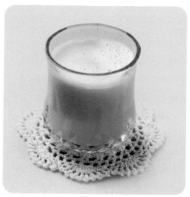

of the pomelo, and peel the white spongy pith off. Remove the seeds and cut into small pieces. ❸ Put the tomato and pomelo pieces into the juicer. Add enough water to juice.

Effects: Tomato clears internal heat and eliminates toxins, cooling the blood and calming the liver. It is rich in lycopene, has a strong antioxidant ability, and can lighten spots and whiten skin.

Broccoli and Cucumber Juice

Ingredients: half a broccoli, one cucumber, one apple, lemon juice, honey

Method: ❶ Wash the broccoli and break into small florets. Blanch with hot water.

❷ Wash the cucumber and cut into small pieces. Wash the apple and cut into small pieces. ❸ Put the broccoli, cucumber, and apple into the juicer. Add enough water to juice. ❹ Add lemon juice and honey to taste.

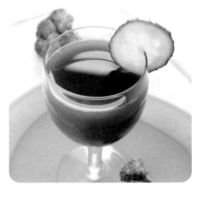

Effects: The rich vitamin C in cucumbers can whiten the skin, maintain the skin's elasticity, and reduce the formation of melanin.

Radish and Olive Juice

Ingredients: one radish, five green olives, one pear, lemon juice, honey

Method: ❶ Wash the radish and cut into small pieces. Wash the green olives. Remove the pits and cut into small pieces. ❷ Wash the pear,

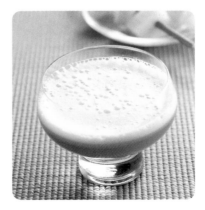

remove the core, and cut into small pieces. ❸ Put the radish, green olives, and pear into the juicer. Add enough water and juice them. ❹ After it is done, add lemon juice and honey to taste.

Effects: Radish moves *qi*, stimulates digestion, moistens the lungs, enhances detoxification, and encourage diuresis. It is also rich in vitamin C, and has a whitening effect on the skin.

2. Life Prolonging Recipes for the Elderly

As a person ages, changes in the body become very noticeable: the eyes begin to lose their clarity, the ears are not so sharp, the muscles start to loosen, and the legs and feet are not as flexible. Therefore, for elderly people who want to try detoxification, the first thing is to ensure a proper diet, so that the nutrients from food can be absorbed to nourish the whole body. The second thing is to keep exercising and not let your body slacken.

Light diet and regular meals: Elderly people who are obese are prone to cardiovascular disease. Therefore, their diet should be light, with a reduced intake of salt. Generally, the daily salt intake of this group of people should be reduced to 5 g, and that of the patients with hypertension and coronary heart disease should be limited to below 3 g. An effective way to prevent overeating and control weight is to keep regular meals in terms of time and quantity of food.

Ensuring adequate intake of protein: This is because the anabolism in elderly people's bodies is reduced, while catabolism is enhanced. The digestion and utilization rate of food protein is decreased. As a result, more protein is needed to supplement the consumption of histone protein.

Appropriate physical exercise: When elderly people who are obese engage in appropriate physical exercise, their body heat consumption will increase. This will encourage fat decomposition, and achieve the goal of detoxification and weight loss. However, the amount of exercise should vary from person to person. Generally, the heart rate of an elderly person should not increase more than 30% after exercise, and there should not be any chest pain or palpitations.

Reducing calorie intake: People with obesity should strictly and permanently limit their calorie intake. They should increase the burning of body fat for detoxification and weight loss. Following a low-calorie, low-fat, low-cholesterol, and low-sugar diet will create a negative caloric balance to reduce weight.

Taking adequate vitamins and dietary fiber: Elderly obese people should make sure that their intake of vitamins and dietary fiber is sufficient. They should take in around 400 to 500 g of fresh fruits and vegetables every day. If they cannot get enough fruits and vegetables to meet their needs, they can eat more coarse grains, beans, and marine vegetables such as kelp and seaweed.

Here are some recipes that can support elderly people's health and help them to live longer.

Corn and Pork Rib Soup

Ingredients: one corn, 500 g pork ribs, two carrots, salt

Method: ❶ Wash the pork ribs, and chop into short sections. Blanch and drain. Wash the corn and carrots. Cut the corn into short sections. Slice the carrots. ❷ Put the pork ribs, carrots, and corn into the pot. Add water and salt. Boil until cooked.

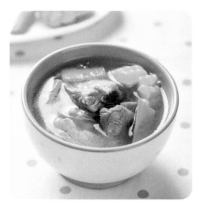

Effects: The rich dietary fiber in corn can moisten the intestines and expel toxins. It is able to reduce cholesterol and prevent common illnesses of the elderly such as arteriosclerosis. Corn also encourages diuresis.

Millet and Longan Porridge

Ingredients: 60 g millet, 30 g longan, brown sugar

Method: ❶ Wash the millet. Remove the pits from the longans. ❷ Put the millet and longan pulp into the pot. Add water and cook. ❸ When the porridge is ready, add some brown sugar to taste.

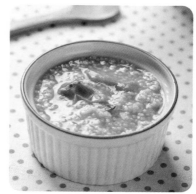

Effects: Elderly people's spleen and stomach can be weak, and their digestion and absorption ability are lowered. Eating food that can strengthen the spleen and stomach, such as millet, can help the body detoxify and strengthen its absorption ability.

Broccoli with Cashew Nuts

Ingredients: 250 g broccoli, 150 g cashew nuts, 100 g carrots, sugar, cornstarch, salt

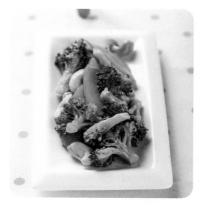

Method: ❶ Wash the broccoli and break up the florets. Wash and slice the carrots. ❷ Blanch the broccoli and carrots in a pot of boiling water. Remove from the pot. Heat the oil in a pan. Add the broccoli and carrot. Stir fry. Add sugar, salt, and some water. ❸ Turn to a high heat. Mix cornstarch with water to make starch. Pour in the starch followed by the cashew nuts. Stir fry and eat.

Effects: The elderly should eat more green food, such as broccoli, mung beans, and cucumbers, to nourish the liver and clear liver fire.

Walnut Porridge

Ingredients: 25 g walnuts, 10 g fresh lily bulbs, 20 g black sesame seeds, 50 g round grain rice

Method: ❶ Wash the lily bulbs, walnuts, and sesame seeds separately. Dry fry walnuts and sesame seeds in a pan over a low heat until slightly burnt. Wash the round grain rice. ❷ Put all the ingredients into a pot. Add enough water and cook over a low heat until it is thoroughly cooked.

Effects: When kidney *qi* slowly enters a state of deficiency, it will not be able to nourish the brain, resulting in the deterioration of the patient's mental ability, speech, and memory. Walnuts can enhance mental ability, tonify the kidneys, and replenish *yang*, as well as strengthening tendons and bones.

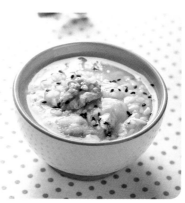

Stewed Mutton with Wolfberries

Ingredients: 500 g mutton, 10 g wolfberries, scallions, ginger slices, cooking wine, salt, coriander leaves

Method: ❶ Wash the mutton. Put the whole piece into a pot of water and cook. Drain and put in cold water. Wash away all the blood foam. Cut into smaller pieces.

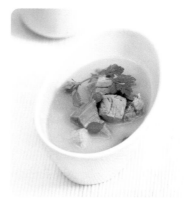

❷ Heat the oil in a pan. Put in the mutton and ginger and stir fry. Pour in the cooking wine, fry thoroughly and then add water to boil. Add wolfberries, scallions, and salt. Remove the

foam from the surface and cover the pan. Turn the heat down and stew until the mutton is soft. Garnish with coriander leaves.

Effects: Lower back tenderness and bodily weakness are the manifestations of kidney deficiency. Mutton can help expel kidney toxins and protect the body from cold.

Celery and Apple Juice

Ingredients: one apple, one stick of celery, lemon juice

Method: ❶ Wash, peel, and core apple. Dice it.
❷ Remove the withered leaves of the celery, and wash and cut into short sections. ❸ Put the apple and celery into the juicer. When the juice is done, add lemon juice. Stir to mix evenly.

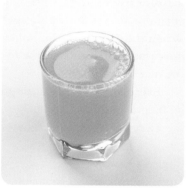

Effects: The dietary fiber in celery is helpful for excretion, while pectin and tannic acid in apples have an astringent effect, and can discharge toxins and accumulated waste from the body.

3. Healthy Growth Recipes for Children

With pollution in the urban living environment becoming increasingly severe, children inevitably accumulate some toxins in their bodies. If the toxins are not discharged quickly, they will have a serious impact on children's health.

Choosing fresh ingredients: Try to choose fresh ingredients, and either boil or stir fry with a small amount of oil. Try not to eat fried food, because it contains carcinogens and damages health.

Cutting down on processed food: Processed food, such as sausages and bacon, is high in sodium. Such food also has high nitrite content, which can cause cancer.

Increasing intake of food that is high in dietary fiber:

In addition to providing balanced nutrition, food that is rich in dietary fiber can also encourage gastrointestinal motility, help defecation, and relieve the burden on the liver and kidneys for detoxification. Fresh organic apples have a good antioxidant effect and can protect cells from free radicals.

Regular bedtime: The human body's golden period for detoxification is from 11 p.m. to 3 a.m. If you can enter a state of complete rest during this period, toxins can be discharged. When the body is resting, blood will concentrate in the important parts, such as the liver and heart, which can accelerate the metabolism.

Exercise: Exercise can support metabolism, boost the flow of *qi*, blood, and fluid, and help the body to expel toxins.

Here are some recipes for children, to ensure healthy growth.

Shrimp Rolls

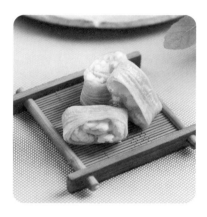

Ingredients: 150 g tofu skin, 300 g shrimps, soy sauce, sugar, sesame oil, salt

Method: ❶ Soak the tofu skin in cold water. ❷ Remove the heads and shells of the shrimps and devein them. Wash the shrimps. Marinate with salt, soy sauce, sugar, and sesame oil. ❸ Put the shrimps on the tofu skin. Roll and tighten. Put the rolls in a steamer for half an hour. Take them out and cut into thick sections when cooled.

Effects: Shrimp is very rich in calcium, which is especially good for children.

Fried Cod

Ingredients: 150 g cod, one lemon, egg, cornstarch, salt

Method: ❶ Cut the lemon into half. Juice one of the halves.

Slice the other half thinly and leave for later use. ❷ Wash the cod and cut it into pieces. Marinate with salt and lemon juice. ❸ Crack the egg, and take only the white. Evenly mix the egg white and cornstarch into a batter. Coat the cod pieces with the batter. Fry until golden. Place on a dish and decorate with the lemon slices.

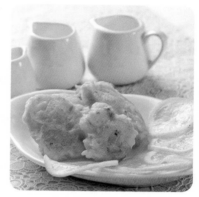

Effects: Lemon peel contains volatile aromatic components that can encourage fluid production, relieve summer heat, stimulate the appetite, and invigorate the spleen. Lemons can increase the appetite, dispel dampness toxin, and invigorate the spirit.

Banana Egg Rolls

Ingredients: two eggs, one banana, 30 g walnuts, tomato sauce

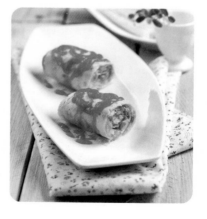

Method: ❶ Peel the banana. Split it into half from the tip. Put the walnuts on each half. ❷ Heat the oil in a pan. When the oil is 50% hot, pour in the beaten egg. Tilt the pan in all directions for the beaten egg to cover it. When the egg solidifies slightly, put the banana and walnut on the egg pancake and roll it up. Continue frying until cooked. ❸ Place the banana egg roll on a plate. Cut into sections. Pour tomato sauce over them.

Effects: The lycopene in tomato sauce is a strong antioxidant, which removes free radicals from the body.

Multi-Colored Porridge with Rock Sugar

Ingredients: 50 g round grain rice, 100 g tender corn kernels, two eggs, 30 g peas, 15 g wolfberries, rock sugar

Method: ❶ Wash the round grain rice and peas separately. Steam the tender corn kernels. ❷ Cook the round grain rice into a porridge. Add the corn kernels, peas, wolfberries, and rock sugar. Cook until they are soft and done. ❸ Whisk the eggs. Pour them into the pot of porridge. When it boils, it is ready.

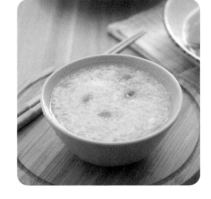

Effects: Corn is rich in dietary fiber, which can encourage intestinal detoxification. It also benefits the lungs, calms the heart, strengthens the spleen, and stimulates the stomach to enhance the appetite, replenishes blood and boosts brain function.

Apple and Raisin Porridge

Ingredients: 50 g round grain rice, one apple, 20 g raisins, honey

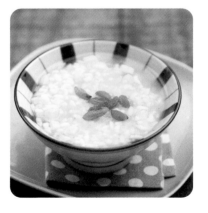

Method: ❶ Wash the rice. ❷ Wash, de-core and peel the apple, and dice it. Soak in water. ❸ Put the rice and diced apple into the pot. Add water and bring to the boil. When it begins boiling, turn the heat to low and cook for 40 minutes. ❹ Add honey and raisins just before eating. Stir to mix evenly.

Effects: Regular consumption of apples can reduce liver and stomach fire, and is beneficial to detoxification. Moreover, apples are rich in zinc, which can boost children's appetite and build up their health.

Strawberry and Honey Milk Shake

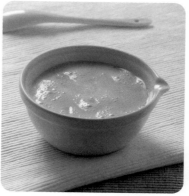

Ingredients: strawberries, honey, yogurt

Method: ❶ Wash the strawberries, and cut into small pieces. ❷ Put all the ingredients into the juicer. ❸ After it is done, pour it out and keep it in the refrigerator for ten minutes.

Effects: Strawberries clear summer heat, detoxify the body, eliminate internal heat, and reduce emotional stress. When eaten with honey and yogurt, strawberries can expel intestinal toxins and boost the appetite. They make very good appetizers.

4. Detox Recipes for Working People

Consumption of rich foods and alcohol is inevitable for people who are often out at social gatherings. Over time, the accumulated toxins will cause serious damage to the body. If nothing is done about it, the liver, kidneys, spleen, and stomach will be damaged to varying degrees. Many office workers remain sedentary for long periods of time, leading to a flabby abdomen. Facing the computer for prolonged periods will also lead to physical issues such as eye pain, deteriorating vision, and dizziness. At work, office staff are advised to stand up and move around every hour. With reasonable dietary detoxification, bodily balance can be restored.

In our daily lives, we should maintain good nutrition and take enough exercise. Our diets should include plenty of water, fruits, vegetables, and grains. Make sure you consume enough cellulose, and eat less high-fat food. Aim for unobstructed bowel movements, and try to maintain a pleasant mood. Get enough sleep so that your body can detoxify overnight. If there is a problem with your liver, lymphatic system, or excretory system, your body's detoxification ability will be reduced.

Stopping bad habits: Avoid going to bed late and getting up late, not defecating in the morning, overeating, missing breakfast, and eating greasy food. Too much greasy or irritating food will produce a lot of toxins during metabolism, increasing the burden on the gastrointestinal tract. Try to use less oil in your cooking. Cut down or cut out fried food. Abstain from eating raw food because it is harmful to the liver. Cooked food should be eaten the same day, not kept overnight. Eat vegetarian food two days a week to give the gastrointestinal system a rest.

Brisk walking: When walking, speed up, and swing and stretch your arms as much as you can. This is a simple way to help your body expel toxins. Brisk walking can help reduce cholesterol and prevent high blood pressure.

Jumping: Jumping can stimulate the lymphatic system to detoxify, help relieve tension, reduce cholesterol, and improve fluid circulation and respiration.

Liver detoxification: The liver is very important for detoxification. In your daily diet, include more carrots, garlic, grapes, and figs, as they can help the liver detoxify.

Kidney detoxification: The kidneys are also important for detoxification. They can help filter toxins in the blood and waste generated from protein decomposition, discharging them from the body in the urine. In your daily diet, include more fruits and vegetables such as cucumbers and cherries, to aid detoxification in the kidneys.

Moistening the intestines and detoxifying: The intestines can help the body expel toxins quickly. However, if you suffer from indigestion, the toxins will remain in your intestines and be reabsorbed, causing harm to your body. Include edible fungus, kelp, apple, strawberries, and honey in your daily diet, as they can help detoxification in the digestive system, skin, and lungs, as well as accelerating metabolism.

The following detoxification recipes are ideal for office workers.

Glutinous Rice and Black Bean Drink

Ingredients: 50 g glutinous rice, 30 g black beans

Method: ❶ Wash the glutinous rice and black beans separately, and soak for four hours. ❷ Put the two ingredients into a soybean machine. Add water and make it into a drink. (If the soybean machine does not have a cooking function, steam the glutinous rice and black beans before putting them into the machine.)

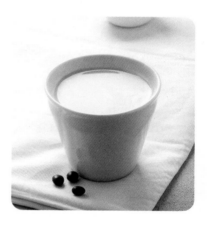

Effects: Black beans are rich in vitamin E, which can remove free radicals and delay the aging process. Moreover, the lecithin in black beans can prevent the production of toxins, avert obesity, and help to maintain body shape.

Celery with Dried Shrimps

Ingredients: 300 g celery, 100 g dried shrimps, cornstarch, scallions, ginger, salt

Method: ❶ Remove the withered leaves from the celery. Wash, cut into short sections, blanch in boiling water and drain. Mince the scallions and ginger. ❷ Heat the oil

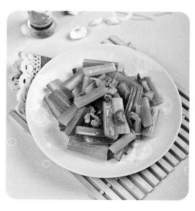

in a pan. Fry the scallions and ginger. Add the celery and dried shrimps, and stir fry for three minutes. Add cornstarch that has been mixed with water. Add salt to taste.

Effects: Celery clears internal heat, detoxifies, lifts the spirits, and reduces swelling, eliminating liver toxicity and lowering blood pressure. It is also effective at balancing a high-fat and high-calorie diet.

Stir Fried Peas with Button Mushrooms

Ingredients: 100 g button mushrooms, 200 g peas, soup stock, cornstarch, salt

Ingredients: ❶ Wash and dice the button mushrooms. Wash the peas. ❷ Heat the oil in a pan. Add the mushrooms and peas. Stir fry. ❸ Add soup stock and boil until cooked. Add cornstarch mixed with water. Add salt to taste.

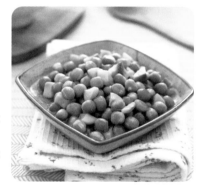

Effects: Peas are rich in dietary fiber, which can prevent toxin deposition. Moreover, the chromium in peas helps the body metabolize sugar and fat. People who socialize frequently should consume this dish for its health benefits.

Peppers with Corn

Ingredients: 300 g fresh corn kernels, one red pepper, one green pepper, sugar, salt

Method: ❶ Wash the red and green peppers, remove the seeds, and dice the flesh. ❷ Heat the oil in the pan, and

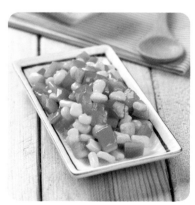

add the corn kernels and salt. Stir fry for three minutes. ❸ Add water and continue stir frying for another three minutes. Add the red and green peppers. Add sugar and stir fry evenly.

Effects: Corn is high in dietary fiber, which encourages digestion and expels toxins, reducing pressure on the spleen and stomach.

Carrot Oat Groat Porridge
Ingredients: one carrot, 100 g oat groats, rock sugar

Method: ❶ Cut the carrots into small pieces. Wash the oat groats and soak them for 30 minutes. ❷ Put the oat groats into a pot, add water, and bring to the boil over a high heat. Turn the heat down and add the carrot pieces. Continue cooking. When the porridge is done, add rock sugar to taste.

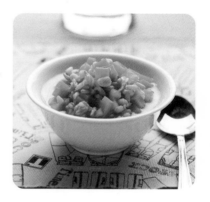

Effects: When eaten often, carrots protect the eyesight, reduce the heavy metal contents in the blood, and expel toxins from the body.

Banana Yogurt
Ingredients: one banana, 200 ml yogurt

Method: ❶ Peel the banana, and cut into small pieces. ❷ Put the banana pieces and yogurt into the juicer. Add water and juice it.

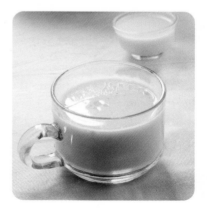

Effects: Bananas clear internal heat and moisten the intestines, and can encourage gastrointestinal peristalsis. The probiotics in yogurt can stimulate the intestines, shorten the amount of time that excreta remains in the colon, and as a result, prevent toxin deposition. After drinking alcohol, banana yogurt can reduce the concentration of alcohol in the blood and alleviate palpitations and chest tightness.

Grape and Honey Tea
Ingredients: 200 g grapes, 30 ml ginger juice, honey

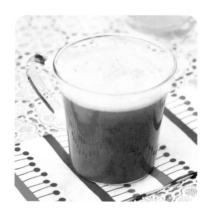

Method: ❶ Wash the grapes. Peel and remove the seeds. Juice the grapes. ❷ Add ginger juice and honey, and mix well.

Effects: Grapes are rich in tartaric acid, which can interact with ethanol in wine, reducing the concentration of ethanol in the body and detoxifying alcohol. Honey can encourage the decomposition and absorption of ethanol, and can alleviate headaches resulting from drinking. Ginger can alleviate vomiting and nausea after heavy drinking. The combination of all three ingredients triples the beneficial effects, and also tastes good.

5. Detox Recipes for Smokers

Smoking damages your own health, and harms the people around you. It also increases the probability of lung cancer and heart disease. Therefore, for everyone's benefit, the best idea is to quit. The following seven kinds of food can help smokers detoxify.

Foods rich in vitamins: There are certain compounds in cigarette smoke that will greatly reduce the activity of trace elements such as vitamin A, B vitamins, vitamin C, and vitamin E, and cause them to be depleted in large quantities. Therefore, smokers should eat a lot of vitamin-rich foods.

Tea: The unique catechins in tea can prevent cholesterol deposits on the walls of the blood vessels. They can also increase gastrointestinal peristalsis, and reduce sugar in the blood and urine.

Foods rich in selenium: Regular smoking reduces the selenium content in the blood. Selenium is an indispensable trace element that works as an antioxidant against cancer. Foods rich in selenium include black fungus, seaweed, garlic, mustard, mushrooms, animal liver and kidneys, seafood, nuts, and egg products.

Foods rich in iron: Smokers should eat a moderate amount of foods rich in iron, such as animal liver, meat, kelp, and beans.

Foods that inhibit cholesterol synthesis: Smoking increases deposits of cholesterol and fat in the blood vessels. When the blood supply to the brain is reduced, it can cause atrophy, and this will accelerate the aging of the brain. Therefore, smokers should eat more food that can reduce or inhibit cholesterol synthesis, such as fish, soy products, and some high-fiber foods.

Nuts and coarse grains: Nuts, coarse grains, and other foods rich in vitamin E can reduce the incidence rate of lung cancer in smokers by about 20%.

Foods rich in β-carotene: Alkaline food rich in β-carotene, such as broccoli, spinach, carrots, pea sprouts, lettuce, and cantaloupe, can inhibit nicotine addiction.

The following detox recipes are ideal for smokers.

Lily Bulb and Lotus Root Soy Milk

Ingredients: 50 g soy beans, 30 g lotus root, 20 g glutinous rice, 5 g dried lily bulbs, rock sugar

Method: ❶ Soak the soy beans, glutinous rice, and dried lily bulbs for two hours. ❷ Peel and wash the lotus root. Cut into tiny pieces. ❸ Put all the ingredients into the soy bean machine. Add water and start the machine. When the soy milk is done, strain and add rock sugar to taste. (If the soybean machine does not have a cooking function, steam the soy beans, lotus root, glutinous rice, and lily bulbs beforehand.)

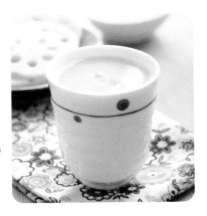

Effects: Regular consumption of lily bulbs can enhance lung function.

Radish with Scallions

Ingredients: radish, scallions, salt

Method: ❶ Wash and cut the radish. Mince the scallions. ❷ Heat the oil in a pan. Add the radish and stir fry. Add water. Lower the heat and stir fry for a few more minutes. ❸ Add salt and continue to stir fry. Sprinkle the minced scallions, and stew for a short while.

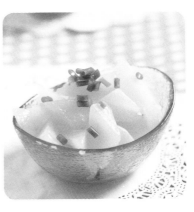

Effects: Radish can encourage digestion, enhance the appetite, accelerate gastrointestinal peristalsis, and support metabolism and the excretion of toxins from the body.

Mango Milk Custard

Ingredients: two eggs, half a mango, 100 ml milk, sugar

Method: ❶ Peel the mango and dice it. ❷ Whisk the egg, add milk and sugar, and mix evenly. ❸ Put the egg and milk mixture in a steamer, and cover with plastic wrap. Bring water to a boil. ❹ Steam for ten minutes and turn off the heat. Remove the plastic wrap, and add the diced mango on top of the custard.

Effects: Mango is good for the stomach, and moistens the lungs. It is very effective at alleviating the discomfort caused by pulmonary toxins.

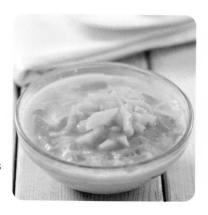

Pumpkin Rice Paste

Ingredients: 100 g pumpkin, 60 g glutinous rice, 20 g raisins

Method: ❶ Wash the glutinous rice. Soak it for more than two hours. ❷ Wash the pumpkin, remove the skin and pulp. Slice the pumpkin. ❸ Put the glutinous rice, pumpkin slices, and raisins into the soybean machine. Add water and select the mixing and cooking function. Dish out and garnish with raisins. (If the soybean machine does not have a cooking function, steam the glutinous rice and pumpkin beforehand.)

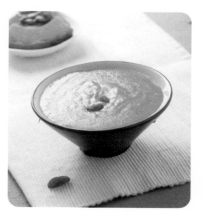

Effects: Pumpkin is rich in pectin, which has strong adsorption. It can bind and eliminate bacteria and toxins, and combine them with excess cholesterol in the body to prevent arteriosclerosis. Regular consumption of pumpkin can relieve asthma, swelling, and lung discomfort.

Osmanthus and Lotus Root with Glutinous Rice

Ingredients: one segment of lotus root, 50 g glutinous rice, maltose, osmanthus syrup

Method: ❶ Peel and wash the lotus root. Wash the glutinous rice, and drain dry. ❷ Cut one of the ends of the lotus root to be used as a cap. Stuff the glutinous rice into the holes of the lotus root. Cover the lotus root with the cap and use a toothpick to secure it. Put it in the pot. Add water to the pot, and make sure the water level go above the lotus. ❸ Add the maltose. Turn up the heat to the maximum, and bring to the boil. Turn the heat down to low and simmer for 30 minutes. Remove and cut into slices. Pour osmanthus syrup over the slices.

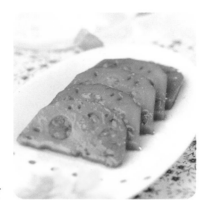

Effects: Lotus root clears internal heat and moistens the lungs, cooling the blood and removing blood stasis. It can also encourage the discharge of waste products from the body.

Loquat and Honey Drink
Ingredients: two loquats, honey

Method: ❶ Wash and peel the loquats. Remove the pits and dice them. ❷ Put the diced loquats into the juicer. Add water and juice the fruit. ❸ Pour out the juice and add honey to taste.

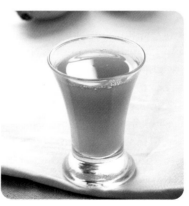

Effects: Loquat dissolves toxins accumulated in lungs and respiratory tract, and can repair the respiratory mucosa. Moreover, the minerals and B vitamins contained in loquats can also support metabolism and improve the body's detoxification ability.

Index